The Compassionate Christ

Spiritual Passwords for Hospital Ministry

By Fr. Larrie Soberano

DEDICATION

I dedicate this book to the loving memory of my beloved brother

Benigno Soberano Jr.

who left this earthly world to join the company of angels

also

to the memory of

Msgr. Artemio Baluma

ACKNOWLEDGMENTS

I would like to offer my sincere gratitude to the following people, for without them I may not have had the courage or confidence to write this book. My encounter with them inspired me to write.

To:

Archbishop Martin Currie, Archbishop of St. John's and Grandfalls Diocese, who brought me here to Canada and inspired me in so many ways; he was my first mentor.

Bishop Richard Grecco, who was an Auxiliary Bishop of Toronto and now a newly appointed Bishop of Charlottetown, Prince Edward Island who also inspired and helped me; he was a strong wall to lean on.

Bishop Richard Gangon, Diocese of Victoria, for his generosity and kindness in appointing me to work in his Diocese as Hospital Chaplain.

Msgr. Michael Lapierre, the Chancellor and Vicar General of the Diocese of Victoria whom I consider my mentor now and help me in so many ways, especially when I was settling in here.

The family of the Couples for Christ and handmaids of the Lord, who help me in my ministry and inspire me in their noble calling, their unwavering service and ministry to the church, for the sanctity and renewal of marriage vows and the importance of family values.

Elizabeth Keefe my good friend, who helped me out editing and proofreading my work.

And last in no means least, to Margaret McGrath whom I consider my surrogate mother here.

I know that to say "Thank you a million times" would never be enough.

CONTENTS

INTRODUCTION

I never thought that I would come to the point where I would write a book, although it came to my mind many times. I had no confidence to put into writing the experiences of life that would I guess, inspire and tells one's story and it never crossed my mind that I would be working as a full time Hospital Chaplain in my ministry as a priest even though I took my (CPE) Clinical Pastoral Education in Makati Medical Hospital back in the Philippines; I thought it just ended there.

I thought it was just a requirement for our seminary formation, but it is not, it happened. I have to accept that time swiftly flies and I have already worked for more than a year as a full time Catholic Chaplain; and that's the fact.

I came to Canada via Newfoundland where I stayed for three years and although I was appointed an Associate Pastor for my first year and became an Administrator for two years, I still worked also as a part-time Chaplain at the hospital, for I was always on call. Upon leaving Newfoundland I moved to the cosmopolitan ministry in the Archdiocese of Toronto where I stayed for two years, again as an Associate and while there I was always assigned to the hospital ministry.

I have so many interesting and challenging stories to tell about my ministry in those provinces and in those Dioceses', but if I try to tell them all, it would make up another book. But on the other hand, I have to thank God for giving me the richness of those experiences in my priestly ministry. In my experience, the most unforgettable ministries I had were when I administered to the sick and poor souls at the hospital. They are such vivid, memorable and fruitful memories.

This book contains a collection of homilies, reflections and stories, as well as Psalm Prayers that I keep in my memory and in my heart. The homilies and reflections are nourishing to one's drooping spirit and they give us instruction, enlightenment and courage to move on. It includes also the Psalm Prayer which I like most and which, besides the Gospel, is the part of the Bible that I always love to read. So, I said to myself, if I have been given a gift to write, I will not miss out that part of the Bible.

Moreover, this book also tells stories of faith and of my encounters with patients; the memory of which, kept on coming back and haunting me until I put them in writing to make them alive where they may serve as light and hope to those people who experience the same kind of stories.

Many times I have rephrased and edited the introduction of this book but I had to keep on changing it to make it real and at the same time fascinating. I tried to make it true in the real sense but at the same time I have to remember the secrecy and confidentiality of people's life's story.

After my six month probationary period, Bishop Richard Gangon, Bishop of Victoria, appointed me as a Chaplain of the Hospital.

My first reaction was a bit mixed. For six years of my priesthood I worked in a parish, either as an Administrator and as an Associate respectively, and therefore I was familiar with parish work and didn't need to adjust myself to that. But working in the hospital is a bit challenging, it is a new field for me and although I was reluctant, yet I took it as a new challenge, a new avenue to widen the gift of my priesthood ministry.

Working in the hospital is not easy but I must say it is a gift that I asked from God during my ordination to the priesthood. Doctors, nurses, priests, volunteers and I as a Hospital Chaplain, work together for the speedy recovery of every patient but at the same time we know that we are just instruments of God's healing hands and we are to tread patiently, tediously and carefully over the wounds and pains of every patient. But still at the end of the day we rely on His great mercy and compassion to provide what would be the best for each and every one of us. I am like a wounded healer, I bring the healing power of Christ, His presence and compassion but at the same time, I also try to heal my own woundedness and pain.

Furthermore, I have seen many patients reading showbiz and fashion magazines while on their sick beds and so I offer another choice for them: I decided to write a book that somehow they can relate to their stories in the hospital. I believe that spending time in the hospital is not only a place for physical recovery but also a moment where we can spend time thinking about life and our relationship with God; recollecting life in the past, how we use the gift of life entrusted to us by God and how we can do better for the remainder of our journey. All this can be done at a time when we can do nothing else except to entrust our life to the attending doctors, nurses and the Chaplain.

This is the moment when we can really feel the weight of our cross, when we feel it is so heavy and tiresome to carry and when there is no one else we can turn to. We ask His help to ease our burden and upon asking His help, our cross becomes His cross, for He took it from us and made it on His own.

This book is written to inspire the life of the patients, their immediate families, relatives and friends as well as those who have experienced confinement and life in the hospital, those who are experiencing it right now and those who in the future who might spend their lives there.

The names of the patients and other matters have been kept secret in order to protect the sacredness, confidentiality and the privacy of the individual person. These stories are of faith, and how the patients and families were able to hang on to that faith to the very end of their journey.

This is also the story of a Chaplain, the wounded healer, who always has the grace to give his own presence and heart to embrace the sick in the name of Christ. It is about the Chaplain, who is always ready to jump up from his bed even in the middle of the night or at the wee hours of the morning, just to be at the bedside of the patients and family members; the Chaplain who is able to unlock the sacredness of the life of every patient, their dreams, stories, family backgrounds, their triumph, the laughter and joy and at the same time, their sadness, their wishes, pains, failures and frustrations.

It is also the story of the Chaplain who witnesses the mystery of faith, death, life, miracles and the mystery that unfolds beyond them.

Yes, indeed, it is the language of the heart and faith that serves as a bridge for myself and for every patient I visit. Through the gift of my priesthood, it is my joy to show the compassionate side of Christ in the midst of their misery, adversity and hopelessness.

Why is the book titled "**THE COMPASSIONATE CHRIST**"?

The first time I met one of the chaplains of the hospital and after she gave me a tour of the different sections, wards, and floors of the hospital, she explained to me the 'dos and don'ts', the privacy requirements and the confidentiality of every matter. Yes, loud and clear I treasure and keep everything in my mind, the sacredness of life and the importance of every story.

After an hour of instruction she then said, "Don't forget the password when you enter in this room; you cannot enter unless you learn the password." She meant the code number to the office of the Chaplaincy and then I said to myself, she was right; to work in the hospital, I have to know the Spiritual Password. I cannot unlock the hearts and stories of the patient unless I know the Password and that Password I created myself, through thorough reflection and incessant prayer. At the hospital, I cannot unlock and enter into the life and heart of the individual unless I learned it, and that Password I share with you.

THE COMPASSIONATE CHRIST—This is a good book to read because in every chapter of this book I give my reflection and it can be used as a resource book for homily materials. In it, I share the joy of my ministry through my writing so that those who want to stay at home can read it when they have nothing to do but to think about the gift of life and their mission in it. The text of this book is not written in highly falloten terminologies, it is written in a very common way and is easy to understand so that not only the scholars and intellectual can understand but it is written so that even a simple mind with a simple educational background can enjoy reading it and at the same time, can reflect on the gift of life. It is more about the language of the heart.

One great philosopher once said: "The heart has its own reason which the reason does not know." and this is it. It is written more in the language of the heart. Jesus thanks His Father in the gospel of Matthew (Mt. 11:25) saying: *"I thank you Father, Lord of heaven and earth, because you have hidden these things from the wise and intelligent and have revealed them to infants."* The wisdom of every page that lies within should not remain in this book; it should be lived out and shared with everybody to complete the meaning and mission of this Password.

COMPASSION

When I was in the seminary, I studied Spanish and Latin for two years, but I must say, it was not enough to know the whole rules and syntax of the Latin and Spanish grammar. We used to decline the noun according to its use and conjugate the verb that always agreed with the subject. There I learned that the word 'compassion' came from two Spanish words, 'con' means "with," and 'passion'—'pasiones' which means "to suffer." The Latin word 'compassion' is from the word 'cum' which means "with" and 'misericordia, misericordae 'which means 'passion'. It is in the feminine gender and belongs to the first declension. This is what I want to focus my idea on, the word 'compassion' which means 'to suffer with."

The word of St. Matthew (Mt. 9 :36) says: *"When He saw the crowds, He was moved with compassion to the depths of His being, for they were bewildered and dejected, like a sheep without a shepherd."* I can really feel the heart of Jesus bursting with so much passion, with so much emotion boiling inside when He saw these people in their pain and in agony. He wanted to ease the pain of these people, He wanted to calm them down but in the subtle and discrete ways that people can best understand and won't be offended. He suffered with what the people suffered.

Jesus was aware that during the time of pain and suffering most people became very sensitive and emotional too. He was so gentle and sensitive to the feelings of others. I remember each time I have to go to the hospital to administer the last rite, especially during the time when I had just woken up from deep sleep at midnight or in the wee hours of the morning. I answer the phone and if it is an emergency call then I should to go to "ahora mismo" as fast as I can and most of the time, the family members are there waiting for my arrival. Or sometimes I have just arrived home from the hospital and am about to take off my coat and clerical polo when the phone rings again for me to go back to the same hospital to do the last rite again for someone else. At first I would get impatient, but when I thought of the importance of the Sacrament to the dying person and the faith of the people who request a priest, and the meaning of my calling, to bring the presence of Christ on them through me, I soon changed my frowning face. I had to go. And the prayer that I asked from God was," Lord change my frowning face into your calming face and let the people see your compassionate side through me."

It is a gift to work in the hospital, it is a gift to journey through the pain and suffering of these people who suffer not only on the physical level but mostly in their spiritual needs. Most of the time, the priest, hospital Chaplain and the volunteers who visit and bring communion bring the best gift they could offer, their gift of presence with their smile and comforting touch. I must say that seventy percent of Catholic patients to whom I administer the Sacrament were seniors and most of the time they could not hear me well, but one hundred percent of them 'heard' me through my smile and compassion which can make your visit worth remembering.

Jesus has a heart that never asks questions; His heart is bleeding to help, to extend the most compassionate word and action He could offer to those who are sick and also to the dying person. He is filled with the great desire to wipe out the tears from every eye, of every patient and also the family members. And this would be the attitude that every chaplain and volunteer should carry to every visit. We bring Christ to them, we bring the real presence of Christ, His love, His acceptance and His compassion; like Him we never ask what sickness a person has, but what matters most is our desire to let them experience that they are not alone, Christ is with them. Christ is not removing their pains and suffering right away but through our presence let them realize that Christ is journeying with them in their pains and loneliness. They are not alone but Christ is with them.

Jesus never looks on our unworthiness and sinfulness with anything but mercy and compassion. He is so connected to every pain and struggle, not only to the people in bed but also for every person who carried their lives so heavily. He was moved to compassion by the world's pain. He was moved with compassion for the sick (Matthew 14:14) and in our afflictions, he is afflicted. As a priest I could tell many personal stories about the difficulties and struggles of every patient in the hospital. When I am taking care of the sick, it seems that I become completely exhausted myself. It seems that I took their illness, their every affliction, their pain and struggle and make them my own. Then, in my moment of silence I usually go to the chapel and throw them away, everything, yes everything, to the oceanic mercy of God.

In my own experience as a priest, I can really feel the hands of God work mysteriously in me as His "Alter Christus' in giving the Sacrament to the sick and the dying. St. Francis of Assisi once said (later quoted by St. John Vianney): "If I saw an Angel and a priest, I would bend my knee to the priest and then to the angel."This is really how the importance of the priest is for those who are about to leave this earthly life and begin their new life in Christ. It is the priest who lets them go and sends them with blessing and prayer; blesses and assures them that the journey is not fearful, and gives them hope to see the light at the end of the dark and seeming endless tunnel. The new light of dawn is waiting for them at their new and permanent home forever. For those who have total faith in God, the priest is a humble bearer of God's compassion and God's healing power. There are times I try to explain why that is but at the very end of the day, I must admit it is beyond my own human power and comprehension; it is just that I become His simple instrument to carry the will He wants for each of the persons in the bed.

STORY

It was early in the morning when I was called in to the hospital to give the last rite; the social worker who attended the family called a Catholic priest to assist spiritually the needs of this family whose faith was being tested. I arrived in the hospital at three in the morning and looked for the ICU, as the patient was in critical condition. He was shot and the bullet went to his liver and close to his lungs. The family members were there, full of tension and anticipation, waiting for the doctor to come out to hear the update on the condition of their loved one. I was with them to spend quality time with prayer and listening to their stories. For a little while they tried to evade their true feelings by telling me stories about how they migrated here to Canada, how they struggle to cope with the demands of living with a difficult culture and the language barrier. But in the back of their mind, I knew they were not at ease, there was something they were anxious about, something was bothering them.

Every time the door of the ICU opened they stopped talking and put their two hands close together hoping that the best result would be heard from the attending doctor and nurses.

The doctor came out and told us that for seven hours they had worked so hard; two doctors and five nurses were attending to him, trying to revive his life but in his condition there was a ninety percent chance that he was going to die. The doctor said "I cannot let you in Father, but I know miracles happen when we pray together and we pray for the best." I thanked God that I was able to spend quality time with the family just with my presence and prayer.

I know miracles happen because after three days the family called me to visit the patient; he as already alert and his brain was working well so I gave him the Sacrament of the Sick and a blessing. After three months I saw the Mom and she was so happy to inform me that her son is doing so well and is now out of the hospital. He had lost perhaps twenty pounds but that was only good for him. He looked different but what mattered most was that he had become more serious about his life. His life had completely changed and I am so happy because he is always looking forward to go to receive the Eucharist every Sunday and I am so grateful to God, for giving him another chance to live. This time we have a life worth living which happened in the name of the Loving God who shows compassion to his unworthy and lost child.

PRAYER
(PSALM 79: 8-13)
Do not remember against us the iniquities of our ancestors
Let your compassion come speedily to meet us
for we are brought very low.
Help us, O God of our salvation.
For the glory of your name;
Deliver us, and forgive our sins
for your name's sake.
Why should the nations say,
"Where is their God?"
Let the avenging of the outpoured blood of your servants
be known among the nations before our eyes.
Let the groans of the prisoners come before you;
According to your great power
preserve those doomed to die.
Return sevenfold into the bosom of our neighbors
they taunted you, O Lord!
Then we, your people, the flock of your pasture,
Will give thanks to you forever;
From generation to generation we will recount your praise.
Amen.

OBEDIENCE

This is one of the two most important, yet difficult, words to observe in an honest way. During our Ordination, we the priests, promise to obey the Bishop for the rest of our lives.

The Bishop asks us, "Do you promise respect and obedience to me and my successors?" then all of the priests answered "Yes," otherwise we did not become priests after all. Another thing we promise is to live the life of celibacy. Obedience and Celibacy are two important things in our life as priests but at this point, I will try to reflect on the virtue of Obedience. Obedience means to obey and follow the church's teachings, particularly our allegiance to the Holy Pope, and to obey our local ordinary, the Bishop. I must say, our discipline and training in the seminary in a way helped in how I appreciate the meaning of obedience in the life as a priest and my ministry.

In the seminary, we were trained to follow rules and regulations. The bell in the seminary played a very important role in signaling the next routine activity such as waking up in the morning, our time at the chapel, time for morning Lauds followed by breakfast and time to prepare ourselves for studies. In the afternoon it signaled time for *"manualia or laborandum"* two Latin words for 'works'. At this time we usually clean the house, from the lobby and parlor to the bathrooms. We also clear the weeds outside in the gardens, cut the grass and plant any kind of trees, making plots for plants and vegetables. Some seminarians were expected to feed the animals like cows, goats, chickens, ducks etc.

We worked usually for one hour every day, but if there was a big event like Family Day or September Fest, there was always an 'open house' when we would invite visitors, parents and benefactors to come to visit us. Usually, seminarians had prepared a special program that would showcase their talents to the visitors. In the evening we had Vespers and if we didn't have mass in the morning, Holy mass will follow after the Vespers. At seven in the evening we were in the dining room for supper followed by recreation which consisted usually of indoor games. At eight o'clock we were expected to be at the chapel for Night Prayer followed by study period and then lights off and total silence. If you stayed beyond that hour you would have to ask permission from the Prefect of Discipline otherwise it will count against your deportment.

Military soldiers live with discipline and order and so it is also in the life of seminarians who are under formation, they are molded and formed for good future priests. This was the schedule that we usually had in the seminary formation:

Monday to Friday
5:30 am—rising
6:00-7:00 am—Mass and morning Lauds
7:00-7:45 am—Breakfast
7:45-8:30 am—Prepare for school
8:30-12:00 midday—School or Library
12:00-1:00 pm—Lunch
1:00-1:30 pm—Siesta
1:30-4:00 pm—School
4:30-5:00 pm—Laborandum/manualia
5:00-6:00 pm—Shower/laundry
6:00-7:00 pm—Vespers
7:00-7:45 pm—Supper
7:00-8:15 pm—Indoor games,

8:15-8:45 pm—Night prayer
8:45-10:30 pm—Study period
10:30 pm—Lights off

Saturday
8:30-12:00 am—Manualia/laborandum
12:00-1:00 pm—Lunch

In the afternoon, we prepare ourselves to go for Apostolate, or we go to the parish and help them with their activities. Usually we taught catechism and joined in Youth ministry. At five pm Sunday we were expected to be in the seminary again. For the entire scholastic years, that is for five years, I lived this kind of schedule and then theological life began with almost the same schedules and activities which lasted for another four years. It is like when the scholastic life (learning about reasoning) ended, the life of faith begins in theology years. We were under formation, we were formed to follow. It is very interesting to know that every priest started from this, following the rules and disciplines. In my own experience I was trained first as a good follower. I do believe that this motivated me to form as a good servant with obedience to the Bishop.

Living within the community was not an easy life, I learned that most of the time, it is not what I wanted but what the community needed that came first. To be a good follower and to listen to the formators would help me somehow appreciate what the meaning of obedience would be in the chosen life I picked. Obedience in the church and to the Bishop is another thing; it is very important in the life and ministry of the priest. It became so challenging to some but for me I saw it from a different angle. For me, obedience is making you free through all privileges handed to you by your Bishop so you may discover the richness of your gifts as a priest, the richness of your diocese and the mystery of tradition that is given to the mother church as well as the link of my priesthood to the Pope and the fullness of my priesthood through the Bishop. Therefore it is not a blind obedience, it is a free willing, a choice that I made for the rest of my life. When the Bishop asked me to carry out the hospital ministry, though I had doubts about my own capabilities, I did not refuse. I tried my best to do what I could, to bring spiritual healing and sacraments to the people in the hospital especially those who are in bed. For me it is a grace and a gift, though I am unworthy; but I was given such tremendous and challenging work to do where I can explore the gift of my priesthood not only in the parish or office work but mostly to the individual person that I use to impart my ministry.

To obey is a gift that you ask from God, without doubt but trusting that He is working side by side with me. To obey is to follow what is the will of the Father, not only for my own convenience and personal agenda but for the sake of the mother church. This is also true to every one of us because to obey is to be faithful to the command of Christ and to observe His laws and decrees. I always believe that the Bishop is the voice of God, the spokesperson, the envoy. He speaks what is the best for us in matters of faith and so therefore, I listen to him and we can ask and have things clarified. We are blessed if we have a Bishop who is very pastoral, has a clear vision and mission for his Diocese for besides the teaching and shepherding of his people, a Bishop who has a compassionate heart or an eagle's eyes, sees the inner needs of his people and is ready to leave His comfort zone just to take care and embrace the wounded sheep in the field; he also has the quality time to nurse and heal them of their pains.

Obedience is a gift that would remind us that we can understand fully the teachings of the church and that somebody will tell us what to do and lead us to a safer way by listening to what is good for us. Working at the hospital I found that most of the senior people had a very strong and solid foundation in their Catholic Faith. At times I was just amazed and wondered at such faith and total submission to the Catholic teaching. Times have changed unfortunately, and seldom do I witness that kind of faith in the young generation of today. It is a privilege and at the same time a gift that I myself experience when I see that their faith is still alive to these senior people whose days on earth can be counted. Maybe the systems of their body become worn and their eyes become dim but nobody would contest their faith for they have it surely engraved from the bottom of their heart. Even to the very end of their life's road, they submit themselves to their faith and their love for our Catholic Church, and that is the most important aspect at the end of one's journey.

STORY

I loved to visit this particular man; he was very happy and all I could see was a man with a big smile every time I visited him in his bed. The lumps that grew around his lips did not stop him from talking and he talked about his active involvement in his parish and how he was an officer of the Knights of Columbus; he was a very nice man, vivacious and full of life. He had been diagnosed with a cancer that had grown inside his throat and on the outer part of his lips grew lumps. He called me to visit him one day because the day after, he was going for surgery and he wanted to receive the body of Christ and to receive the Sacrament of the Sick. I visited him. I introduced my name and my position in the hospital and he was very delighted that a Catholic priest was available right away to journey with him and to listen to his stories.

He was about seventy five years old and ready to face the great challenge of life. He told me that in his lifetime he never missed the church service especially Sunday mass and that in his own simple way he was following the teachings of the Catholic Church. He talked about celibacy, for he is a single and he had no regrets about his chosen vocation and is really happy as a single man. After my first visit, his smiling face really registered on my mind and I then realized that I had encountered such a wonderful person who, in the midst of his adversities, had a wonderful life to share. The next day was Ash Wednesday and after my mass, I visited him again to bring him the Sacred Ashes as I did to all the Catholic patients in the hospital. I also went to let them know that the season of Lent had just begun so that they can reflect on the mystery of the salvation, through reflecting the life, passion and death of Christ while at the same time connecting their crosses to the suffering and pains of Jesus on the cross.

On my way to his ward I was surprised he was in the living room watching TV and he still tried to smile in spite, of the bandage which covered his lower lips where the doctor had removed the lumps. I saw stitches around his mouth but still he was amazing, and he was so happy that he had received the ashes. He told me that he was grateful for the wonderful gift of life and he enjoyed it very well. In his own humble way he is going to follow and obey what would be the challenge of life ahead of him. Obedience for him is to be happy in following the word of Jesus.

The third time I tried to visit him but he was already out of the hospital. I prayed for his speedy recovery and I pray now that his remaining years of his life will inspire the people whom he knows about the joy of being with God, even though it is difficult to follow His command, especially when things go wrong. Though I brought him the comforting words of Jesus, His presence and His Sacrament, this man brought new meaning to my ministry. I had never seen a big smile from a person whose life was going so much downhill. I was so happy to meet him and I know there are lots of people like him whose faith was tested but their obedience to follow the words of Jesus never diminished. I pray that his life will bring healing to those who don't appreciate the gift of life.

PRAYER
(PSALM 119: 105-112)
Your word is a lamp to my feet
and a light to my path.
I have sworn an oath and confirmed it.
to observe your righteous ordinances.
I am severely afflicted;
give me life, O Lord, according to your word.
Accept my offerings of praise O Lord.
And teach me your ordinances.
I hold my life in my hand continually,
but I do not stray from your precepts.
Your decrees are my heritage forever;
They are the joy of my heart.
I incline my heart to perform your statutes
Forever to the end.
Amen.

MERCY

"Kyrie Eleison, Christe Eleison, Kyrie Eleison." This comes from the Greek word used to invoke God for mercy, that is; *"Lord have mercy Christ have Mercy, Lord have Mercy"* This is the most humble prayer we hear every day at the beginning of the Holy Mass; it is setting the tone of the whole rite of the mass when we beg for mercy. That's what we are, unworthy people, sinners, guilty of all the flaws and selfishness, of masquerades and pride, of brokenness and emptiness inside. By acknowledging our wrongdoings we become naked in front of our merciful God but, He will not exercise his justice for every mistake we make, but will take care of every wound of our spirit and body and heal them by His own love and mercy. We beg the mercy of God to look upon us and shower us with His forgiving presence. He looks on us with so much mercy and love, so much devotion and care, and invites us to enjoy His presence at His banquet. He stays with us for so much quality time to let us know that His heart bleeds for mercy for those who come to him and ask for it.

In the book of the prophet Jeremiah (14:7-10) it says: *"Although our iniquities testify against us, act, O Lord, for your name sake; our apostasies indeed are many, and we have sinned against you. O hope of Israel its savior in time of trouble, why should you be like a stranger in the land like a traveler turning aside for the night? Why should you be someone confused like a mighty warrior who cannot give help? Yet you, O Lord are in the midst of us, and we are called by your name do not forsake us."* When we have nothing to turn to, especially in times of confusion and

27

distress, we turn to God, not as the last resort but anytime. Our lives would be empty without His presence and only in God who always has time to listen to our pleas and petitions and only in God does our wounded soul take rest. He is ever faithful to the very end.

I myself, rely on the great mercy of God. I know very much that I am not worthy to become a priest. I feel that I have nothing in me that I would consider as exceptional traits or skill, but He chose me and blessed me and for that I am very grateful. He did not look on my human failings, loaded with so much vanity and shortcomings. He called me out of his great mercy. I still remember the prayer of the Bishop during our ordination to the priesthood. After the Rector of the Seminary presented us to the Bishop with some inquiries, the ordaining Bishop would say, *"We rely on the help of the Lord God and our Savior Jesus Christ, and we choose this man, our brother, for priesthood in the presbyterial order."* Out of His great mercy and help He chose and consecrated us, His priests, so that through us, His great mercy and help will be experienced by the people in need.

In (Psalm 86: 15) says: *"But you O Lord, are a God of merciful and gracious, slow to anger and abounding in steadfast love and faithfulness."* The mercy of God is overflowing and endless. It never runs out. His mercy is like the ocean you can see where it begins but we cannot see where His mercy ends, for it has no end. In the hospital I have seen a lot of great mercy from God which continues to be present and available to those who want it. If all people value the meaning and the importance of confession, they will share the joy of our Heavenly Father. Confession is not only telling our bad and sinful stories, our sham and shame but also experiencing the great mercy and compassion of God; His loving embrace and joy. God is making us holy and once again making us whole through forgiveness. God will fix what is broken within through His grace and in spite of our brokenness and wretchedness He always has the time to nurse us, and to heal us.

But on the other hand, forgiveness comes to us when we repent. The way to the restoration of God's original creation is repentance. It is when the transparency and humility lays down the sinful ways of who we are and the grace of forgiveness will come to us. When we return home with sincere repentance and receive God's embrace and forgiveness we are restored to our original beauty, our oneness with God. When that reconciliation happens, when we received the absolution from the priest, it is then that God's original purpose is being restored and we can really feel the joy of our Father, whispering like a gentle breeze or chirping like humming bird down there at the bottom of our heart. The joy of the Father and our own joy becomes one and it is the reason to celebrate.

Moreover, God never stops; His bountiful mercy goes out searching for the lost one to restore to the original and wholeness of His creation. He never stops and is always waiting for anyone who wants to 'come home'. It is the joy of the merciful Father to be able to welcome a sinner coming home, because He is full of mercy and compassion. (Mt. 18:12-14) says: *"What do you think? If a shepherd has a hundred sheep, and one of them has gone astray, does he not leave the ninety nine on the mountains and go in search of the one that went astray? And if he finds it, truly I tell you, he rejoices over it more than over the ninety-nine that never went astray. So it is not the will of your Father in Heaven that one of these little ones should be lost."*

STORY

Many times I visited this lady. She was 83 years old and always had a lovely smile. She was a reflective and quiet type of person but her silence spoke a lot about her personality and faith. She always had a rosary in her hand and never missed to pray her devotion to the Blessed Virgin Mary. One time I visited her and she was delighted to introduce me to her best friend, also an older lady. They were neighbors and living in the same apartment building and they were telling me about their life stories, how they shared their lives and how they coped with the different kinds of challenges of old age. Her best friend brought her a lovely rose plant, blooming and beautiful, and there was a message, "Get well soon, my best friend." She was very delighted to receive the body of Christ and the Sacrament of the Sick and we also prayed one decade of the Sorrowful Mystery together with her friend and we offered a prayer for her a speedy recovery. It was indeed a very memorable visit.

When I was about to leave, a patient adjacent to her bed asked me to say a prayer for her also. She told me that although she was not a Catholic, she believed that God is universal and God is for her also and that she wanted to receive a prayer and a blessing too. She told me that she hoped that someday, regardless of religion, we will become one, for we have only one God and we are all created in His image and likeness. It reminded me of the mercy of God that He gave to the gentiles, the republicans, the tax collectors, prostitutes and to a sinner like me. One of the most beautiful parables in the Gospel was the encounter of Jesus with the Syrophoenician woman who had great faith. In the Gospel of Mark (Mk 15: 24-30*)* it says*: "From there He set out and went away to the region of Tyre. He entered a house and did not want anyone to now He was there. Yet He could not escape notice, but a woman whose little daughter had an unclean spirit immediately heard about Him, and she came and bowed down at His feet.*

Now the woman was a Gentile, of Syrophoenician origin. She begged Him to cast the demon out of her daughter. He said to her. "Let the children be fed first, for it is not so fair to take children's food and throw it to the dogs." But she answered Him. "Sir, even the dogs under the table eat the children's crumbs." Then He said to her, "For saying that, you may go-the demon has left your daughter." So she went home, found the child lying on bed, and the demon gone." Yes indeed, the mercy of God is not exclusive to certain people but it is universal and for all.

PRAYER
(PSALM 51: 1-5)
Have mercy on me, O God,
according to your steadfast love;
according to your abundant mercy
blot out my transgressions.
Wash me thoroughly from my iniquity
and cleanse me from my sin.
For I know my transgressions,
and my sin is ever before me.
Against you, you alone I have sinned,
and done what is evil in your sight,
so that you are justified in your sentence
and blameless when you pass judgment.
Indeed I was born guilty,
a sinner when my mother conceived me.
Amen

PRAYER

When the Prophet Elijah fled for his life from the hands of the slaughterer Jezebel, he journeyed for forty nights and forty days to regain his strength at Mt. Horeb, the mountain of the Lord. At that place he came to a cave and spent the night there and in that cave Elijah met God.

In Kings 19:11-12 it says: *"He said "Go out and stand on the mountain before the Lord, for the Lord is about to pass by." Now there was a great wind, so strong that it was splitting mountains, and breaking rocks in pieces before the Lord, but the Lord was not in the wind; and after the wind an earthquake; but the Lord was not in the earthquake; and after the earthquake a fire; but the Lord was not in the fire and after the fire a sound of a gentle breeze. When Elijah heard it, he wrapped his face in his mantle and went out and stood at the entrance of the cave."* God did not reveal His divine presence in the powerful and overwhelming attractions but He revealed it instead in a tiny, gentle breeze. In the silence of our hearts like a gentle breeze, the will of God is revealed for us but when we are busy and there is no silence around us, we then miss the passing of the Lord. Like the Prophet Elijah we need sometimes to withdraw from the hustle and bustle of our lives go to a place of more stillness, solitude and quietness. Only in God does our spirit find rest peacefully. Prayer is communicating with God and we can air our sentiments but at the same time, we must listen to Him through contemplating and meditating. Anthony de Mello wrote "Prayer is kind of like having a vacation with God." We enjoy being with Him, and enjoy listening to what is the best for us in the stillness of our heart.

In the Gospel of Mathew after Jesus had fed the five thousand people (Mt. 14:23) it says:

"and after He had dismissed the crowd, He went up the mountain by Himself to pray. When evening came, He was there alone." Jesus had a very intimate relationship with His Father. After He performed that great miracle, He withdrew from the crowd to spend time with the Father in a very intimate way. I believe that Jesus is telling us that through our prayer, we are invited to develop our intimate relationship with His Father, to spend time in a place where we can be alone with God, where there is no noise and distractions. It is very important to develop our prayer life, to entrust everything to His care, because we don't know what lies ahead of us and the only person who knows what will happen in our journey is Him. And when in any time that our boat is rocking, we will hear His voice saying, *"It is I, do not be afraid."* (Jn. 6:20).

Prayer is our daily spiritual bread, not only for priests and religious people, but also for all of us as Christians whose strength and capability rely on His bountiful goodness and mercy.

I could not find the right words to define the meaning of prayer based on my own experience or even find a word to describe it eloquently but I must confess, prayer is the best invisible weapon I have as a priest that no other people can see; only you and Him. It is like a diamond sword that has a blade at every angle and is placed at the center of my heart; sharp and shining so that at anytime I can pull it out to use. It is an invisible weapon that can conquer any danger along the way, and will serve as my shield and protection. It can slash my enemy and can destroy any kind of vices and any temptations that may be bothering and pestering me. It can soften the heart, can change a person, can change me; can change us. It is very powerful yet, invisible.

Sometimes, some people are not aware that it's there standing at the sanctuary of our heart. They just don't realize it because they never use it; it is when you often use it that it becomes sharper and shinier. Some people cannot see that it's there because they seldom use it, and sometimes, instead of cleaning that space to make it visible, they dump their garbage and rotten waste there so that when they need it most, they cannot use it right away because they still need to clean it up and sharpen it, and that takes time. They still need to remove the waste and dig it out because their heart is where the prayer lies and it has become the dumping place of garbage.

In the Gospel of Luke (Lk. 11:1-4) it says: *"He was praying in a certain place, and after he had finished, one of the disciples asked him, "Lord, teach us to pray, as John taught his disciples." He said to them, "When you pray, say: Father, Hallowed be Your name, Your kingdom come. Give us each day our daily bread. And forgive us our sins, For we ourselves forgive everyone indebted to us. And do not bring us to the time of trial."* The first part of the prayer, "Our Father, Hallowed be Your name" is the part I really like most and for me, I would rather refer to this part of the Lord's prayer than to explain the whole theological meaning of it.

Every time I recite that prayer, it seems that my heart is so intent to say a million thanks to God but those million thanks are not enough for all the gifts He has showered upon me. Yes, prayer is first of all to be grateful to the Father for He is the reason why I am here and I have this beautiful and fruitful life. I begin with Him and I will end with Him but one thing is important, at the end of my day I have to praise and glorify His name in every moment of my life. It is a beautiful world to live in as St. Therese of the Child Jesus would say, "Everything is grace."

In the Gospel of John (Jn.10:10) it says: *"I came that they may have life, and have it abundantly."* As a priest, I have a lot of mistakes and shortcomings, sinner as I am. Many times I cried because I had just missed the opportunity to take advantage of the many things that life can offer but I have no regrets, I am just a simple priest trying to live out faithfully and fruitfully, the calling that I have chosen. I don't have an overly comfortable life, for priests most of the time live alone in solitude, and sometimes if you can't appreciate the life that you have chosen, some priests become lonely and depressed and then some move away from their priesthood and find comfort in a married life. Our priesthood should be anchored with so much prayer and total trust to the providence of God, His grace and many blessings. I am very happy that in spite of my unworthiness He called me and anointed me, and called me as one of His disciples. The only regret I may have when the time comes is that I will be old and cannot serve as well as I am serving Him now, while still His people will be full of energy and inspiration.

For me, my whole life is a thanksgiving prayer because I have nothing to ask for; I would say I am a spoiled son of God. Many times I have blundered and many times I was unfaithful to my calling but still I can feel His faithfulness all the time. I had a lot of challenges in my life, ups and downs, thick and thin moments and many times I failed and I cried, but again, everything is under the wings of the love of God. His grace is enough for me. Surely my whole life is a prayer; a prayer of praise and thanksgiving to the loving Father. We always give thanks and praise God no matter what happens along our journey and with His presence, He always completes our stories and they always have a happy ending. He is good to us and His love endures forever.

STORY
I still recall the smile and the calmness on the face of that lady whom I visited in the hospital. That midnight I went to the hospital and as usual during the night, all the doors are usually closed, so I had to pass through the Emergency Room and most of the time the nurses and doctors were very busy and I have to wait. Usually I approach one

of the attending nurses and say that I have come to visit a certain patient in a certain building, and usually the security guard would escort me until I found the floor and the patient. When I got to the right place I asked the nurse if I could visit the woman and they knew I was coming because the patient asked them to call me. What surprised me was her smile and the joy within her; she was so calm and peaceful. She asked for the Sacraments of Confession, Anointing of the Sick, and Holy Communion. She was so honest when she told me her situation; her doctor had told her she had stage four cancer of the uterus and it had already metastasized to other parts of her body, but what kept her smiling was that the strong faith she had in Him.

The second time we met each other was when she was already dying and could only whisper her words. I went to the hospital at one o'clock in the morning when she was asking for me to hear her Confession, give her the Last Rites and a small particle of the Body of Christ. I explained to her that although it is only a small particle, the substance does not diminish, it is still the body of Christ. She was catching her breath with many medical machines attached to her body. Her husband and her son were there too and were trying to keep their feelings in control although I could see their face full of tears which kept running from their eyes. The moment was so fragile and emotional, so moving that I tended not to talk but to empathize with the feelings that they had.

After giving her the Sacraments she needed, I told her to just give me a call in the morning and I'd come and pray again. She said before I left, "No, Father, this is the last time we will see each other." Then she thanked me for everything, especially the gift of my presence that I gave to her during the time she needed most to be listened to. She said that she will pray for me and hope that I will be happy serving the people here in this Diocese, especially sick people here in the hospital. In the morning after praying my morning Lauds, I drove to the hospital just to see what happened to her. I went to her room and asked the nurse how she was doing. The nurse told me that just ten minutes after I had left in the night she had passed away.

Death is always a mixture of pain and relief. I was happy because she is now at peace, she will not experience so much pain and suffering anymore but at the same time, she was too young to die. On my visits to her I learned many things; she was so strong and she was never afraid of death. She understood very well the meaning of Christian death and she was so prepared and knew she could not hold on to the life she had here on earth. She had an amazing faith and I really admired her for that, because in spite of her situation, she was very thankful for her life. She thanked God that for fifty years, she was blessed with a good husband, a son, a daughter and grandchildren. She was so happy to leave this place and you could see on her face the joy within and the calmness of her spirit. I do believe that when her family bid goodbye to her, they did so in the company of angels and saints, and being the righteous people they are, in their hearts they were rejoicing to have had a very good mother sharing in the banquet of our Savior. At the end of the day, The Lord gives, the Lord takes away. Blessed be His name for his love endures forever.

PRAYER
(PSALM 54: 1-7)
Save me, O God, by your name,
and vindicate me by your might.
Hear my prayer, O God;
give ear to your words of my mouth.
For the insolent have risen against me,
the ruthless seek my life;
they do not set God before them.
Surely, God is my helper;
the Lord is the upholder of my life.

He will repay my enemies for their evil.
In your faithfulness, put an end to them.
With a freewill offering I will sacrifice to you;
I will give thanks to your name, O Lord, for it is good.
For He delivered me from every trouble.
Amen.

ALWAYS AVAILABLE

From my own point of view, the priest is always available to minister to the people, where ever he is and whatever he is doing. I never use the words "It's my day off." or "I'm not available." nor do I ever use my day off as my right or my excuse not to do the sacramental thing asked by the people. Parish work is very laborious, the mass every day, the meetings with different religious groups, consultation and planning with the finance and parish council, attending the sacraments (especially the confession), the weddings, funerals, baptisms and preparing homilies, especially every Sunday and special occasions of the church. Sometimes they are called to visit the hospital especially if the patient belongs to his parish and so I do understand the priest needs to have rest, and that a day off is really sacred to them; they need rest to recharge their batteries. But on the other hand, the life of the priest is more of a mission. We never look at how much we are being paid every day, we look more at how we used the day in fulfilling our calling as a priest. In spite of the busy schedule most of the priests are happy and very contented in the life they have chosen.

Very seldom can I count on my fingers the times I have heard the priests complain of too much work; most of them have inner strength and power and so much enjoy the life they have chosen. Working in the hospital is a bit different, I work for twenty four hours a day and six days a week and always with an ear and an eye to the cell phone. But sometimes I have worked seven days and twenty four hours a week if some priests are not available. I never complain although I also need to recharge my batteries and regain my strength and energy. Working in the hospital is more complicated; the people come and go and I can't really develop my own community. I give them sacraments for a period of time and suddenly after a few days or weeks they are gone. I make rounds in the two hospitals; I bring Communion to the sick and spend a little time talking with them. After my visits I would go to the seashore just to relax and throw away all the negative energy that I had absorbed from the hospital. When I see the ocean, that is how I imagine the love and compassion of God, endless, no boundaries, always there, faithful and waiting.

Most of the time, the ocean is quiet, serene and full of mystery. I stay there looking at the blue water with the sea gulls flying overhead, enjoying the beautiful weather, the sun shine, the fresh air and the beauty of nature while in the quietness, while I commune with the silence of nature, I already have recharged my batteries. I leave all my baggage behind. But sometimes, the ocean is kind of rough; you can hear the noise in the air the roaring of the waves coming to the shore. The sea gulls and the boats seem to be hiding, trying not to see the angry ocean but for me it seems that the ocean takes all my anger, pain and worries and then it gets angry on my behalf and vanishes in to the shore. Spending time by the ocean is a healing time for me. In my own experience I have found the ocean to be therapeutic for both body and mind and it even revives and heals my drooping spirit. When I see the ocean, it is then I reflect that no matter whether it rains or shines, every time I visit the ocean, it is still there, always available to give me comfort, recharging my batteries and allowing me to throw away my negative feelings. It is the ocean that reflects all the healing power of the love of God, His compassion and care are always available, His faithfulness is eternal and He never runs out of mercy and love.

Priests should always be available to administer to the spiritual needs of the people, the requests are many and they should never run out of life-giving water to give to those who are thirsty for the word of God and his forgiveness and gift of presence. I pray always that my fellow priests would go the extra mile to help out the people in need of spiritual help, even if sometimes it means that they have to sacrifice their day off.

STORY

This man has no name for he doesn't know his name. He is sixty six years old and he has been in that building for almost one year. He was admitted in almost the same month as I did my first week of ministry as the full time Chaplain of the hospital for Catholics. I found his name on the list of the Catholic patients but he lived in a different building and because I was new I still had to ask the information person to give me direction to that building. Every time I went to that building I never I found him in his room because he was always moving, always on the go, roaming to and from different places. When the nurse found him and told him that the priest was there to visit him, no matter what he was doing, he would stand up and always have the time to pray with me and receive Communion. Yes, he might forget his own name but the signing of the cross on his forehead registered within his soul so much that he never forgot to do it at the beginning and at the end of our prayer. I could hardly understand him, sometimes even a single word was hard, but his actions of faith, tells everything. He is a man of faith, pure and simple. His mind was demented because of old age but his faith was never touched by any kind of disease like a disease that gradually cripples and kills the body; his faith was untouched.

As human beings, when we have a doubting faith and are experiencing this kind of situation, we have the tendency to evade and to deny what happens to us. Many times we blame other people and things and even God for allowing us to undergo such challenges like this. Sometimes, we become paranoid and bitter; what we see is a glass half empty and we are gloomy from the harsh realities of our experiences. But not this man, not this person, he has a solid faith. He always has the time and availability to be in the presence of Christ and always has the time to pray when everything is wrong. He hangs on the gift for support, and that gift is the gift of faith; that's the gift no one will take from him. That is for me, the most precious gift you own and you bring it and you offer it when this pilgrimage on this earth is through. In spite of what happens you run your race and keep your faith to the very end.

This is also the word of St. Paul on his 2nd letter to Timothy (2 Tim. 4:7) it says: *"I have fought the good fight, I have finished the race, I have kept my faith."* He never really knows that every time I make rounds at the hospital I try to visit him also in his building, not because I have to but because of the faith he has and his humbleness to receive it in his heart and soul; his faith is true and simple. He keeps his faith to the very end and I do believe, if we hope for the best we will still have a lot of years to journey together in the hospital. Our journey of faith is a testimony that Jesus is alive and when everything gives up on our body, we still have a reason to live because our faith tells all; for He lives among us.

PRAYER
(PSALM 46: 7-11)
The Lord of hosts is with us;
the God of Jacob is our refuge.
Come, behold the works of the Lord;
see what desolations He has brought on the earth;
He breaks the bow, and shatters the spear;
He burns the shields with fire
"Be still, and know that I am God!
I am exalted in the earth."
The Lord of hosts is with us;
the God of Jacob is our refuge.
Amen.

SACRIFICE

From the two Latin words 'Sacro & sacra' which mean 'sacred & holy', and the verb 'Facio facere, feci, factum' which means 'To do, or to make" and therefore the word 'Sacrifice' means 'To make holy, or to be sacred'. When I heard the word 'sacrifice', the first idea that came to my mind is Jesus, He died for us as a sacrifice for the salvation of humanity. He gave His life freely because of His unconditional love for us. A very holy and sacred act He did for us, the ones undeserving of His love. In the gospel of John (Jn. 15:13) it says: *"No one has greater love than this, to lay down one's life for one's friends."* The victory of love over all the powers of darkness, of hatred and division, of violence and war is the sacrificial love of the Father, that He gave His only Son. When we see the cross it reminds us of the unconditional love of God; His love is faithful even to the very end.

In our life, when we encounter turbulence and chaos it is then that we make it a sacrifice and an offering to Him; we become one with God and it purifies and sanctifies us. Gradually through prayer and faith we gain wisdom which is the meaning of the cross and hardship in our life and gradually we understand our cross as we connect to the cross of Christ. In the Old Testament we heard the great story of Abraham and Isaac and about the sacrificial love of their long awaited for son, who was born when Abraham and Sarah were well-advanced in their years. The old yet faithful couple finally had their baby whom God had promised to them. However, God spoke to Abraham (Gen. 22:2) saying:*"Take your son Isaac, your only son, whom you love...and offer him up as a holocaust."*

Because of the obedience of Abraham to the word of God, He blessed him. Out of this sacrificial willingness, Abraham becomes the father of all nations. From Abraham's faithfulness, demonstrated by his willingness to sacrifice, comes the blessing of the all the people who believed. In (Gen. 22:16) it says: ***"Because you have done this, and not withheld your son, I will indeed bless you, and I will make your offspring as numerous as the stars in heaven and as the sand as the seashore. And your offspring shall possess the gate of their enemies, and your offspring shall all the nations of the earth gain blessing for themselves, because you have obeyed my voice, "*** This story of Abraham and Isaac's sacrificial love is the pre figuration of the sacrificial love of God the Father and His beloved Son, our Lord Jesus, who gave his life freely for the atonement of sins.

In (Jn. 3:16*)* it says***:"For God so loved the world He gave his only Son, so that everyone who believes in Him may not perish but may have eternal life. "*** And at the same time, the same sacrifice is made present at the celebration of the Eucharist. His life, death and resurrection, is made present in the sacrifice of the Holy Mass. It is the sacrificial love that saved us from damnation. In our day to day experience, any sacrifices we have in our life that we do in the name of love and faith in God, are precious and glorious and anything that we offer as a holy and sacred act denotes many blessings from God. When we do something good, we forget any interest owed for the sake of the love of God and his people, and that is what we call it sacrifice.

Sacrifice is self giving, self emptying and it is always what you can offer best to those people in need without expecting any compensation and not waiting for anything in return. It is dying of oneself that we can find something worth remembering in our life as a good Christian. It is in doing good to others, that we find lasting happiness and life. I do believe we have a daily sacrifice, and that is Jesus is telling us, "If you want to be my true disciple, take up your cross, deny yourself and follow me." People in the hospital have a lot of sacrifice to bear. Most of the sacrifice they keep inside their heart and this sacrifice has no meaning at all, until we connect it to the life of Christ. His cross reminds us every day that He is always with us and that by bearing our cross every day, our life story becomes more sacred and holy. In (1 Peter 4:12) it says: *"But rejoice, insofar as you are sharing Christ's sufferings, so that you may also be glad and shout for joy when His glory is revealed. "*

STORY

I still remember the presence of this couple whom I visited when I started my ministry in the hospital. The woman was diagnosed with cancer, and the husband was there almost all the time, every time I visited her. Unfortunately, after living for thirty years as a married couple they were not able to produce children on their own but I have seen on their face the quiet and calmness of entrusting their life to God; for He knew the reason why they didn't have any children of their own. Yes, I visited her many times. She had a soft voice and was a very pious woman. I was not sure how old she was, but I guessed around sixty or something. The first time I visited her, she was sleeping and the husband was there. I talked a little while to the husband and I learned from him about the goodness and kindness of his wife When she was still healthy and active, he told me, his wife was the 'jack of all trades'. She could do everything in the house, from marketing, carpentry, gardening and cooking and she was a very good cook too; she was indeed a super woman. Since the doctor found that she had a brain tumor, after she fell down, her health had deteriorated and gradually she became sickly all the time; she could not do the things she did before. It seemed that half of her body became paralyzed and she was lame and crippled. He tried to do what she had been doing, because of his love and caring for her. She did everything for him before, but now he does everything for her too.

I must confess that he was a devoted, faithful and loving husband and he was there after his work to see his wife all the time. I prayed for them, especially for his wife who entrusted her life to our Creator, the Giver of Life and the best Physician, the Wounded Healer (who is Jesus Christ) had; and we prayed together, entrusting her life to Him. When I was about to leave, she woke up and I introduced myself to her and she told me to stay for a little while. She was a nice lady and the husband would look at her lovingly and always held her hand; they are indeed a nice and good couple. I asked her how much she loved her husband in spite of the fact that the husband looked tired and haggard. She looked at her husband and said "My husband completes me and I complete him and we could hardly live without each other." I was stunned with that powerful answer. The love was so pure and real, so brave and everlasting. But the sacrifice of the husband was there at the very beginning and he was faithful to the very end.

I visited the wife many times but she was slowly deteriorating and what was vivid to my mind, was the teary eyed husband looking to his wife with love and care while at the same time, he was powerless and cannot help her in that situation. What a sacrifice on his part; a sacrifice that perhaps defines the meaning of love between these two. Love is their sacrifice. They both promised to God and his church to live together through richer and poorer, in sickness and health, till death do they part but I do believe they will continue to move on, and hold on to that faith. As they lived out their promises, Jesus was also making promises to walk with them; to walk with us until the end of the world. As we reflect the words of Jesus. In (Mt. 28:20) it says: ***"I will be with you till the end of age."***

PRAYER
(PSALM 50: 14-50:23)
"Offer to God a sacrifice of thanksgiving,
and pay your vows to the most High.
Call on me in the day of trouble;

I will deliver you and, you shall glorify me.
Those who bring thanksgiving as their sacrifice honor me;
to those who go the right way
I will show the salvation of God."
Amen

SERVICE

There is a beautiful song that goes: *"We are made for service to care for all men,*

We are made for love, for time and again, The love that will make through sorrow and pain The life that will never die with strain." It is a beautiful and meaningful song that really defines what it means to be of service. The word 'deacon' comes from Greek word 'diakonos' which means 'servant or waiter'. In the Catholic Church we have two kinds of Deacons, namely a) Permanent Deacon and b) Transitional Deacon The candidate for the Permanent Deaconate who is married must have reached thirty five years of age and have the consent of his wife (Canon 1031[2]). An unmarried man must not be admitted to the Permanent Diaconate unless he is twenty five years old, and has manifested a desire to remain unmarried (Canon 1031[2] and 1037). In accordance with Canon 87 the local ordinary, who is the Bishop, could dispense from the age requirement within his territory for a just cause for a period up to one year (Canon 1031[4]).

Chief among the faculties accorded to Permanent Deacons is preaching the Word of God. Canon 764 states that a Deacon possesses the faculty to preach everywhere, to be exercised with at least the presumed consent of the rector of church. Second Vatican 11 Lumen Gentium (no. 29) lists the faculties which may be granted to a Deacon: to administer the Sacrament of Baptism solemnly, to be custodian and dispenser of the Eucharist, in the name of the church to assist at and bless marriages, to bring the Sacrament of the Sick to the dying, to read the Sacred Scripture to the faithful, to instruct and exhort the people, to preside at the worship and prayer of the faithful, to administer Sacramentals and to officiate at funeral and burial services.

There are two great deacons of the church who stand as great pillars to our faith. The first is St. Stephen. His feast day we celebrate on December 26th. He was the Archdeacon and Protomartyr, the first martyr as he was on trial and being persecuted. St Stephen experienced a theophany. His theophany was unusual in that he saw God the Father and the Son:

"Behold, I see the heaven opened and the Son of man standing on the right hand of the Father (Acts 7:56). The second one is St. Lawrence. His feast day falls on August 10th. He was one of the seven deacons of the ancient Rome who were martyred during the persecution of Roman Emperor Valerian in the year 258. He was placed in charge of the administration of church good and care for the poor. During his torture, Lawrence cried out,"This side's done, turn me over and have a *bite.*" In Latin it says *"Assum est, inquit, versa et manduca."*

Yes, indeed these two great deacons spread miracles and conversion to many. The church has honored them, and gave them special feast days to remember them. Transitional Deacons on the other hand, are one step before becoming a priest. He must be a celibate man who intends to become a priest and vows to obey his local ordinary (the Bishop) and the whole church. Every priest passes that stage. Our priesthood is anchored with service, we are called to serve, not only the priest or deacon but every Christian is called to serve.

Priesthood or Holy Orders is the Sacrament by which men become priests and are given a sacred power (sacra potestas) to act in total sacramental identification with Christ (i.e, to act in persona Christi) in order to confect Christ's Body and offer it up to the Father at the Mass for the remission of sins; to forgive sins through the Sacrament of Penance, to solemnly Baptize; to preside during the Sacrament of Matrimony; to offer Unction to the dying; to preach; and to otherwise teach, guide, and sanctify their sheep. With, and only with the permission of the Bishop, he may be delegated to offer Sacrament of Confirmation, but to the Bishop alone is reserved the power to ordain other priests. As in Baptism and Confirmation, the Sacrament of Holy Orders leaves an indelible mark on the soul of the recipient and can never be repeated once validly received; once a priest, always a priest (even if a priest is laicized and removed from his office, this mark remains). As said, the minister of the Sacrament of Holy Orders is the Bishop, and the matter of the Sacrament is the imposition of hands, which takes place during the beautiful ceremony of ordination. The form of the Sacrament is the words: ***"Grant, we beseech Thee, Almighty Father, to these Thy servants, the dignity of Priesthood; renew the Spirit of holiness within them, so that they may hold from Thee, O God, the office of the second rank in Thy service and by the example of their behavior afford pattern of holy living."***

The Bishop on the other hand has the greatest authority and jurisdiction (aside from the Pope and Patriarchs) and has the power to ordain men into the diaconate and priesthood, and to offer the Sacrament of Confirmation, though this last power they can delegate to a priest if necessary. He is said to exercise the fullness of the priesthood. Deacons, Priests and Bishops are the three majors in the hierarchy of the Sacred Orders that are meant to be for the great service for the glory of God. In the Gospel of Mathew (Mt 20: 26-28) it says: "But whoever wishes to be great among you must be your servant, and whoever wishes to be first among you must be your slave; just as the Son of Man came not to be served but to serve, and to give His life for the ransom of many."

As the late Mother Teresa of Calcutta once said, *"To serve is power."* It gives you an opportunity to see what the human heart can be capable of, especially for those who are powerless and destitute, deprived and poor and lonely. We can make a different kind of service, where we have something to offer that can bring hope and make a difference in the life of a person, and uplift the dignity of life. Service is priceless. You are not expecting anything in return, or doing something you expect a reward for. It is an overflowing kind of kindness and generosity that comes from your heart; that is, the heart of every person patterned to the Sacred Heart of Jesus, There is nothing to keep but always only to give. I have encountered people who give service to the parish, and expect no amount of compensation in return, they devout their life in the name of God. They never expect anything in return and they want to help the priest in planning and in serving the people of God in their own little way. Jesus gives His love in the name of service. When we give service, that's a power; the power of how far the heart of human being is capable of doing good to his less fortunate brothers and sisters of Jesus. In the Gospel of John (13:12-15) it says: *"After He had washed their feet, had put on His robe, and had returned to the table, He said to them, "Do you know what I have done to you? You call me teacher and Lord— and you are right, for that is what I am. So if I your Lord and Teacher washed your feet, you also ought to wash one another's feet. For I have set you an example, that you also should do as I have done to you."*

STORY
There are so many ways that we can make a difference to this world out of our selfless love; we call it service and I have seen and encountered lots of people who have extended the life of others because of their devotion, generosity and kindness. Lay people or active parishioners who share their treasures, talents and time for the betterment of their church, especially those who are involved in the

financial needs of the parish and the pastoral council who work side by side with their pastor for leading and serving their community. We also hear about a lot of rich and famous people who have different ways to extend their help to the people who are deprived of education, healthcare and quality of living.

On the other hand I have seen also people whom I considered as servers of God to the sick people at the hospital, residents of retirement homes. They are volunteers who untiringly bring Communion to the sick every Sunday and for me, I think they are noble and an example to give service with a cause. These people not only bring the Body of Christ to those who are sick but with their mere presence, they also journey with the pains and struggles of the lonely and sick people. For me they serve as crutches, spiritual friends of those people who need help to awaken their spiritual needs. They are people who have golden hearts. These people work behind the scenes and are committed to bring the presence of Christ to those who are down trodden and worried. They offer their very self, without waiting for any kind of favor or anything in return.

In my mind one woman stands out. She was a retired nurse and she had a very happy family, loving and understanding husband and three daughters who already had their own families. She was blessed with so many things in life and she returned it by giving service to sick. She came every Friday and Sunday to bring Communion to the sick and to listen to the inner thoughts of sadness and loneliness of these sick people in the hospital. I really admired her and the rest of the volunteers who were always there to take care of the spiritual needs of the sick people.

Working at the hospital is not easy, sometimes the Chaplain and the volunteers had to wear gowns, gloves, and masks if the patient is in isolation and we take also a risk, just to do the meaning of service. But in spite of that, this lady is very happy doing what she is doing; she has been satisfied and fulfilled for so many years doing these things and she would do it again and again for her love and service, especially to the sick people. Her service to the hospital is a way of thanking God for His gifts to her and her family. And I believe these volunteers working at the hospital, are also called by God to give service to the sick in a very special way. For me, they live out the very meaning of service in their lives.

PRAYER
(PSALM 100: 1-5)
Make a joyful noise to the Lord, all the earth.
Worship the Lord with gladness;
come into His presence with singing.
Know that the Lord is God.
It is He that made us, and we are His;
we are His people, and the sheep of His pasture.
Enter the gates with thanksgiving,
and His courts with praise.
Give thanks to Him, and bless His name.
For the Lord is good;
His steadfast love endures forever,
And His faithfulness to all generations.
Amen

INSTRUMENT

I still remember the 1995 World Youth Day that was held in the Philippines. I was still under formation then and was in my first year of theology. It was indeed one of the most memorable events that happened in my life's journey. I was so blessed and fortunate to be a part of that big event; it was an euphoric feeling when I saw the Pope riding in his bullet proof Pope-mobile. I was approximately three meters away from where he was, and for me, I must say that it was really rewarding and consoling and it gave meaning and inspiration to my calling to priesthood.

I saw the jubilation of most people trying to glimpse the face of the Pope during that time. The theme song of the 1995 World Youth Day is still fresh in my mind "Tell the world of His love." It was so mesmerizing and that song I can still sing by heart; so moving and meaningful. That's why I wanted to start my reflection with that song, that we are all instruments of God's love.

Yes, first and foremost we are instruments of spreading around the abounding love of God and tell of that abounding love throughout the world. God wants us to tell the whole world about His love, tell those people who live in darkness, those people who have never experienced the real essence of love, people who are broken, who are shattered, lonely and hopeless. Tell that the love of God brings healing, a promise of a new beginning and new hope for those who want to experience this love. We are all instruments to rekindle that love in their broken hearts and we are called to make it happen. The beautiful song of Hosea in the Catholic Book of Worship 11 says:" **Come back** *to me with all your heart, don't let fear keep us apart, Trees so bend though straight and tall, So must we when others fall.* "This is one of my favorite hymns during the season of Lent. The love of God is haunting us and is always looking for our coming back home where His love protects and embraces us, where His love serves like a comforting blanket. Through this I can feel that the loving kindness and loving mercy of God is so close to us; closer during the season of Lent. When I tried to find the parallel of this song this is what I found.

In the book of the Prophet Hosea (6:1-3) it says: *"Come, let us return to the Lord; for it is He who has torn, and He will heal us; He has struck down, and He will bind us up. After two days He will revive us; on the third day He will raise us up, that we may live before Him. Let us know, let us press on to Know the Lord; His appearing is as sure as the dawn; He will come to us like the showers, Like the spring rains that waters the earth.* " There is a certainty in the love of God to His people; like the certainty of dawn that scatters the darkness of night or the refreshing gift of spring rains that bring new life. Just like the sun that brightens the day and breaks the darkness, so the love of God scatters every fear and every doubt from the heart of every person.

The love of God is so faithful and it never ends. The word "**hesed**" means His faithful love; His steadfast love is everlasting even to his faithless people. The merciful love of God is meant to be shared with those who never have it, to those who live in the dark corners of the world. It shall not rest from us. What God asks from us is to be an instrument to share with others the gift we have received from Him that we are meant to give away. I have seen many patients to whom God has given the gift of his loving mercy and kindness, though most of them confessed that they don't deserve another chance, but God has given them another opportunity. That's how the love of God works, it creates wonders and miracles. It brings new life to them that they have never had before; a life that is filled with so much love and compassion from a loving God and because of their encounter of that "*hesed*," they too are ready to share the life they have, to inspire other people. They are now the instruments of God giving healing love to others and they become their life giving spirit. I believe that most of the nurses and doctors, chaplains and volunteers feel it is not the duty that they wanted to fulfill at the end of the day that counts most, but the gift of love they wanted to share to every patient they encounter. And we want to pass it on.

STORY

We are all instruments of God who serve and praise His name through serving the needs of his less fortunate brothers and sisters. Working at the hospital I've seen a lot of people try to extend the life of the patient. The family members and friends are always there to comfort the sick, most of the time they give inspirational stories, moments of laughter and good experiences that would remind them of their happiness when they were together with the patient. They are the ones who know the back ground, the ups and downs of the person. They are very blessed if they have immediate families and friends around who would always be there at their bedside every time, especially in the moments of loneliness and nostalgia about the life she or he left behind. But sometimes, when I see the old people who are at the hospital where I work, there is no one around except the doctor, nurses and hospital Chaplain who work tediously to bring back the life of the sick person. They are the three persons who would always be there to journey through the down moments in the life of the patient.

The doctors and surgeons, who have noble professions, dedicate themselves to protect and save the lives of the individual sick person to the best of their abilities. They are always there to do whatever is needed. Their time for the patient is precious, for they have to attend to the physical needs not only of one person but for the others who need a surgeon and doctor's advice. Indeed, all of us rely on the findings of the doctor for our physical health; a noble and delicate profession worthy of respect and praise. Though the doctor is the one I look up to, I would rather give credit to all the nurses, and nurses' aides who work at the hospital and different home care houses for they spend more time at the bedside of the patient. I oftentimes have connection with them, talk to them and even establish friendships with some of them. I know both of us are aware that in many ways we have common encounters with the patients at the hospital.

I interviewed one of the nurses about her profession. She told me that it is more than a job, it is more than the salary she received, it is about calling, it is a vocation that at the end of the day, it is not how much she was paid, but it is the life that is worth living and which is rewarding. She is very happy with her profession and taking care of the sick is her passion. And she said, if she was given another life and a choice what kind of profession she will take, she still would choose the same profession, a nurse. She told me about the hardship also as she found the night shift was challenging and if she is on duty, she had to be extra careful, especially monitoring the sick persons who were assigned to her. Another one, is dealing also with family members who are sometimes overwhelmed with the patient critical condition and need extra care for their feelings. All the time the nurses were always there to check on every one and also the physical dynamic of the patient. Besides her family, to whom she is committed to being faithful and loving, the next is her profession; that is, taking care of the sick to the best of her abilities.

She told me also, that if it happened that a patient died on her time of duty, the really hard part is to explain to the family members all the things that she needs to explain, but the most devastating part is when she becomes attached to that person. She would have to talk and see to the patient, take their temperature every day, then, the person finally gives up their life and was gone. She said "When you take care of the sick, most of the time you put your heart unto it but that is what I have to do, and it is part of my calling."

The other nurse I interviewed is already retired after serving for forty one years in that noble profession. What she remembered most were the moments of happiness that she spent during her life at the hospital and with the patients. She had no complaints but had to thank God for this profession which allowed her, together with her loving husband, to send their children to school, to provide everything they needed, and now they have become professional too. Because of the inspirations she had shown to her children, three of them now are also working at the different hospitals. She told me that she did really enjoy her life at the hospital and she committed herself to the best of her abilities and now she deserved to take a break and enjoy the life she missed. She had a lot of stories to tell about her experiences at the hospital; she always had a smile and laughter to share. Indeed she was one of the pioneering instruments of God's saving hands to those who were sick at the hospital here in this Diocese. Beside the doctors, the nurses are also deserving of our respect and gratitude for they serve as God's instrument to save, and take care of the sick brothers and sisters of Christ.

PRAYER
(PSALM 89:1-4)
I will sing of your steadfast love,
O, Lord, forever;
with my mouth I will proclaim
Your faithfulness to all generations.
I declare that your steadfast love
is established forever;
Your faithfulness is as firm as the heavens.

You said "I have made a covenant with my chosen one,
I have sworn to my servant David:
I will establish your descendants forever,
And build your throne for all generations."
Amen

ON CALL

"On call." I often heard these words from the mouths of the nurses and doctors, and I know that it means they are on duty for twenty four hours straight. Even though they are enjoying the company of family or friends in their homes, at anytime they may have to make an exit and go in to the hospital to attend to the physical needs of the patient. The idea of being 'on call', was not really clear to me until I experienced it myself as a full time Catholic Chaplain at the hospital. The first few months I really enjoyed the hospital work, it was new to me and I felt that I had found my inner joy in serving the sick. I really appreciated the joy it brought as it became clearer and clearer that this is my life, this is my calling, this is what God wants me to be for a period of time.

When I'm on call, first of all I have to check if the cell phone is recharged and loud enough to hear when it rings. I have to bring the cellular phone wherever I go as I have to be vigilant, always waiting for the calls, because any moment it may ring. I remember one time when I was invited to the party after a baptism. I was about to start eating when my cell phone rang and the nurse asked me if I can come as soon as possible for any moment the patient will pass away and the family members were there. At first, I was thinking 'Why did they always called the priest at the last minute, I was in the hospital yesterday and they never phoned me and now I'm here at the party and I was about to enjoy my food and meet some good people, and now they expect me to go.'

Well, what could I do but go and carry out my ministry; this is why

I'm here as Chaplain in the hospital. Sometimes I miss the calls but they always leave a message in my voice mail and if it is from the hospital it is announced as "Private' and no number appears for returning the call so then I have to call the operator to find what hospital they called me from.

To work in the hospital can be uncomfortable because of the unpredictable calls because if I am 'on call' I cannot go away from the city because I have to calculate that my driving will not take me more than an hour away from the hospital. If I only think about my own pleasure and interests I believe I can't be a good hospital Chaplain; I have to set aside my interests and put the 'on call' of my ministry first, where it will be my priority and my happiness. The Parable of the Good Samaritan Luke 10:30-37 says: *Jesus was telling a parable: "A man was going down from Jerusalem to Jericho, and fell into the hands of robbers, who stripped him, beat him, and went away, leaving him half dead. Now by chance a priest was going down that road; and when he saw him, he passed by on the other side. So likewise a Levite, and when he came to a place and saw him, he passed by on the other side. But a Samaritan while traveling came near him and when he saw him he was moved with pity. He went to him and bandaged his wounds, having poured oil and wine on them. Then he put him on his own animal brought him to an inn, and took care of him. The next day he took out two denarii gave them to the innkeeper and said, take care of him, and when I come back, I will repay you whatever more you spend. Which of this three you think was a neighbor to the man who fell into the hands of the robbers?" He said "The one, who showed him mercy." Jesus said "Go and do likewise."*

The priest who is also the Chaplain of the hospital is always a kind of a good Samaritan; always on call, always on the go, always ready to sacrifice his own comfort just to attend to the spiritual needs of the sick and the family requesting it. The hospital Chaplain is about love and a life worth dying for, the service of a wounded traveler and wounded people. He must forget what he likes and what he is doing for a moment just to bind tediously the wounds and give his helping hands to those who are crippled, old and fragile. It says in the gospel of Mark (Mk. 6:45-50 *after Jesus fed the five thousand: "Immediately He made His disciples get into the boat and go on ahead to the other side, to Bethsaida, while He dismissed the crowd. After saying farewell to them, He went up on the mountain to pray. When evening came, the boat was out on the sea, and He was alone on the land. When He saw that they were straining at the oars against an adverse wind, He came towards them early in the morning walking in the sea. He intended to pass them by. But when they saw Him walking on the sea, they thought it was a ghost and cried out; for they all saw Him and were terrified. But immediately He spoke to them and said "Take heart it is I; do not be afraid."* Jesus was always leaving His own interest and was always there for some kind of rescue. He was praying with the Father on the mountain top but when He saw the disciples had trouble with the strong wind, He forgot His comfort and went off to help them. What matters most for Jesus is putting that prayer into action; the faith should be lived out and shared with those who needed it most.

STORY

After making rounds from the two hospitals, usually my routine in the afternoon is to try to go for walk or go jogging and one of my favorite spots is to Sea Side Walk where I can see and touch the scenic ocean. I usually run for one hour and stay for a little while to feel the therapeutic site. On one instance I was called during my running and the nurse told me to be there as soon as possible. I told her to tell the family members I'll be there around fifteen or twenty, for the place where I was, was not really far from the hospital. I usually brought extra clothes, my clerical polo and things that I needed every time I'm on call and I put them in the back seat of my car as I can't even travel farther than one hour's drive away from the hospital. When I arrived I asked the nurse about the patient and she told me that the family members were waiting inside. I came in and four of them were crying, trying to put the oxygen on the mouth of their mother who was eighty eight years old. She still heard us and was awake but couldn't speak. The son told me that during her healthy years his mom never missed the mass; her life in the mornings included attending mass every day. But since she was crippled and wasn't able to go by herself, she stayed in their house and volunteers from the parish brought her Communion every Sunday. She was a very active and pious woman, who had a devotion first to God who provided everything, then her husband who had died five years before and then to her loved ones. The son told me that the doctor gave her twenty four hours to live and they were asking for the Sacrament of the Sick and prayers for the whole family. We prayed together and we sang the Salve Regina.

What inspired me so much is their love to their mother, even the grandchildren who stayed outside the room because they was not enough place inside, were crying. I saw in their eyes the love and care they had for their grandmother whose life was on the brink of death yet they still hung on to their faith, a faith instilled in them by their grandmother. I was consoled and rewarded when I saw the faith of the people and how they tried to put the importance of faith before their struggle and worries. No matter what I was doing in my own personal interest when the call comes I have to attend and just be there in their midst to bring the healing oil and the prayer, to journey with them through their difficult moments. So is the life of the Chaplain; I leave everything behind when the call is on. Many times I was called to bring the Sacrament of the Sick during my deep sleep in the wee hours of the morning and to be there with the grieving family members to bring calm and peace to them and also to read the consoling words of Jesus Christ in the Gospel; this is the challenge of this ministry. It is unpredictable, yet always I have the gift of my presence for those who want to receive the healing power of Christ. My joy is when I see the faith of the person and his family members and their humility to accept things that are really beyond their power; the total surrender to the care of the One who Gives us life. When I see this faith in people, my joy is complete.

In the book of James 5:13-17 it says: *"Are any among you suffering? They should pray. Are any cheerful? They should sing songs of praise. Are any among you sick? They should call the priests of the church and have them pray over them, anointing them with the oil in the name of the Lord. The prayer of faith will save the sick, and the Lord will raise them up; and anyone who has committed sins will be forgiven. Therefore confess your sins to one another, and pray for one another, so that you may be healed. The prayer of the righteous is powerful and effective."* Yes, indeed, the priest is an extension of God's healing hand to give compassion and healing power to those who ask and believe in His name. The priest will continue to do the ministry and give hope, restore faith and bring the message of Good News to these down trodden people in their bed.

PRAYER
(PSALM 4: 1-8)
Answer me when I call, O God of my heart!
You gave me room when I was in distress.
Be gracious to me and hear my prayer.

How long, you people, shall my honor suffer shame?
How long will you love vain
words and seek after lies?
But know that the Lord has set apart the faithful for Himself;
the Lord hears when I call Him.

When you are disturbed do not sin;
ponder it on your beds, and be silent.
Offer right sacrifices,
and put your trust in the Lord.

There are many who say, "O that we might see some good!
Let the light of your face shine on us, O Lord!"
You have put gladness in my heart
More than when their grain and wine abound.
I will both lie down and sleep in peace;
For you alone, O Lord, make me lie down in safety.
Amen.

NEW

The well known New Testament is also called the New Covenant of our Lord and Savior Jesus Christ. The word Gospel is from the Anglo-Saxon "Godspell," meaning good news. Ultimately the word comes from the Greek 'Euangelion', also meaning good news. The word 'Gospel' can mean the Good News of salvation preached by Jesus Christ, or the Good News preached about Jesus. Every day we read the Word of God many times, but when we start reflecting on it again, it can offer different meanings; it is like a diamond which points to different angles of our life, it always gives new meanings and points of view. It is the same with life, as we try to live the Word of God in our humble little way. Although I go in and out of the building of the hospital almost every day there are times when it feels new to me. I always encounter new people, new patient's names on the Catholic list, and this is something that I always have to embrace and take it as a challenge.

Every time I make my visit, I must say, something new happens; new insight, new reflection and new experiences making a new person happen within me. Even the nurses and doctors change their shifts every now and then, and this means I have to introduce myself again and again. Visiting the hospital always brings me new discovery and wisdom to ponder. It is very fruitful, because I bring the healing power of the Sacraments, the Oil, Confession and the Body of Christ, to the patients for healing both body and soul. Staying in the hospital for a few weeks or even a few days, for the sick people changes something within.

I know how difficult it is to be a patient in the hospital because I had my own share of pain staying in the hospital for few days after my diaconate ordination. I had a fever and was over fatigued, and at the same time my final oral "revalida," the final oral exam at the seminary, had just happened. I know how the people in the hospital feel, I was counting the days till when I got out and every time the doctor made a visit I prayed that there was nothing else to find in my body, or any another sickness or symptom that would force me to stay in the hospital; there is no place like home. Because of that experience I want to be careful with my health and I want to take care of my body because waiting for the results of my medical and physical tests made me sick with worry and unrest.

That experience brought me new realization that I have to take care of my body and at the same time, be able to empathize with the feelings of the people in the hospital. I can really connect my life to them in their awkward situation, their longing to get out. Their world becomes narrow and limited but I do believe that once they get out from the hospital, something happens to them, they know now how to value the virtue of waiting, being patient and embracing survival. They know also that people, no matter how strong and healthy they are, may at any moment find themselves being confined in the hospital and we don't really have one hundred percent assurance that our bodies are well. An accident happens when you are in a most unguarded moment and sometimes an accident or a casualty is caused by another person or nature. Life is full of surprises. It always offers new horizons, new avenues and good news for us to savor the mystery and fruitfulness as life unfolds.

As a Christian, when we trust our life to Jesus, He always offers new meaning, new hope and a new beginning. I know that every wound and the scars that are left on our body, are a sign of the love of God; God still holds on to us and he does not want us to let us go, He is always begging us not to give up, He is always giving us many chances that maybe we can change our life for better. Those marks and scars on our body are the hands of God, He has a hold on us and we are in a kind of tug of war, between Him and death. He gives us a time to reflect and to value the sacredness of our lives, while we can do nothing only remember Him and remind Him that only He can do something for us. He wants us to love Him, to love Him with all of our heart, all of our soul, and with all of our minds. He wants us to love with the whole of our being; not partially and not mostly of our selves. He is asking from us the totality of that love. In the midst of our nothingness, when we are unable to do anything when our body is relying on medical machines to keep us alive, we can think of Him. We can rely on Him because we know He can do something far beyond what we would expect. He works on the inner healing which comes first, and so when you experience the pain of physical woundedness, you have nothing to worry about. When we entrust our whole life to Him and only Him it gives new meaning and offers a new beginning to us, and if it is His Will to give us another privilege, the privilege to continue to live here in this world, we have to be grateful. If He decides to take us from this world He will take care of us and we will encounter the love and peace which we had never had when we were here on earth and we will find peace, serenity and contentment in His presence.

STORY

I still remember a certain lady who was ninety years old and whom I used to visit the hospice many times. I really enjoyed her stories and her smiling face. She stayed in the hospital for six weeks and was excited to go home because she told me that her son who lived in Alberta was coming for his wedding, to be held here in Victoria. It was a second marriage for her son as his first wife died many years ago. They planned to visit her in the hospital before the day she was scheduled for discharge and she told me, "I feel I've become older here in the hospital. Before my son sees me, I should be looking new, wearing something new, something fresh. I am scheduled today to go to the beauty parlor, and to see my hair stylist. I don't want my son and his wife to see me like this. My hair! I never had hair like this." After few weeks she called me to visit her apartment and she asked if I could bring the Sacrament of the Sick and if she could receive Holy Communion. I found her very happy and contented. She said "Father, there is no place like home; I'm here." she said. She was so delighted to tell me her story about the wedding of her son I saw that she was indeed new; she told me that once a week her hair stylist comes to fix her hair. I believe I see a glow in her eyes and in her spirit and that is something new which she learned from staying in the hospital.

Indeed, coming out from the hospital, restored not only our fractured pieces of our physical parts but mostly our broken spirit. Yes, she was new; she was not wearing the hospital gown anymore and sleeping beside another patient. She is different now and looking out over the veranda, I can see the lovely budding rose, with green leaves and other plants around. They are also happy that this lady came home and be with them for a second time around. I can see the sunlight and the beautiful panoramic view of the city, where she lived. It is indeed a new life for her, a new beginning. Every day brings new hope and opportunity to appreciate the beauty of life. I pray this time, she would be very careful with her health and enjoys the remaining years of her life.

PRAYER
(PSALM 67: 1-7)
May God be gracious to us and bless us
And make his face to shine upon us,
That your way may be known upon earth,
Your saving power among all nations.

Let the people praise you O God;
Let all the people praise you.

Let the nations be glad and sing for joy,
For you judge the people with equity
And guide the people among the earth.
Let the people praise you, O God;
Let all the people praise you.

The earth has yielded its increase;
God, our God, has blessed us.
May God continue to bless us;
Let all the ends of the earth revere him.
Amen.

ALPHA

In the Book of Revelation 22: 13, Jesus said: *"I am the Alpha and Omega, the first and the last, the beginning and the end."* Alpha is the first letter and Omega is the last letter in the Greek Alphabet and it is very interesting to know that Jesus declares himself, as the first and the last, the beginning and the end, and we believe. During the Easter Vigil, when we Catholics and other Christians who celebrate the paschal mystery of Christ life, His Passion, Death and Resurrection, there is a moment at the beginning of the ritual when all the lights are turned off, and then there is the Blessing of Fire at the entrance of the Church. There is a big paschal candle to be lit from the fire and it is interesting to know that there is a big cross shaped in the middle of the candle and the hole that Jesus was nailed into. On that cross also is written the two words, Alpha and Omega. These symbolize that we, as Christians, begin with Him and end with Him.

From that Pascal candle we light our own candle as the priest and cantors walk up to the altar. That Paschal candle stands there in the sanctuary at the beginning of Christian life and also it is a witness when our body rests inside the church at the end of our Christian life. The Paschal candle is used during our Baptism, where the godfathers, and godmothers light their candles as witnesses to the entrance of every baptized child into the Catholic church. It is also stands tall during the funeral mass to give the light for the last time and to signify that we were born out of light and we will surely end in that light. All the seven Sacraments we receive from the Catholic Church as we begin to embrace the name after Him and we receive every now and then, the many graces and blessings from Him as sons and daughters of God. When persons are baptized, they are dying with the original sins we inherit from the great fall of Adam and Eve. But in that first Sacrament we also rise to a new life, a new beginning in the life with Christ. We are no longer captives of sin but become heir to His Eternal Kingdom. The indelible mark, the sign of the cross that the priest or deacon put on our foreheads testifies that we begin in the name of Christ and when everything is through on this earth's journey the cross in our tomb bears a living witness that once as we lived as Christian, we also died as a Christian.

When persons receive the Sacrament of Reconciliation, they have chosen the welcoming embrace and loving kindness of the Father. They choose life and despise death and they open their hearts and received the bountiful grace of God for the new beginning of relationship.

When persons receive the Sacrament of Matrimony, they are dying to a single self and begin to live as co -creators of God to subdue the earth, where love and family are formed as a new beginning of relationship with God. When persons receive the Sacrament of Confirmation, they are starting a new life of solid and mature faith, strengthened by the gifts of the Holy Spirit. When a person receive the Sacrament of Holy Orders, they are dying with their selfish interest so that they can begin a new life with service and ministry in God's vineyard.

When we receive the Sacrament of the Eucharist, we are being renewed by making present the life of Christ, His life, death and resurrection here and now. When persons receive the Sacrament of the Sick, they are given the grace to endure their pains and their sufferings but also they are being prepared for a new life that is about to begin, a life that will reveal everything, where death becomes powerless; but a new life will spring out that is eternal with God.

The Seven Sacraments always give us dying of oneself but at the same time create a new beginning of relationship with Christ. Yes, we begin our life story and we end our life story with Christ; he gives our life and he will take away from us, for we are not the owner, we are just a caretaker of our life. That's why no matter how much we hold on to that life, we can only pray for the best, but we know that the life we have has a real owner. We are all transient of this world, we will never travel this way again and each one of us will have the privilege to meet Him and tell our own story and we hope and we pray that our story starts and ends with him. It is really challenging to explain to the family the meaning of our faith during the death of their love ones. As a Chaplain I will show how my faith works, that in the silence of our heart, we know that He is taking care of the one who gives. No matter how much we try to give that love to a person who dies, there is a greater love, greater than we give to that person, a love that is beyond imagining, a love that human persons cannot give, a love that is unconditional. We cry because our loved one dies, but we know that they are very contented right now because they are a person who was searching for the true meaning of love, and finally they found it through the loving embrace of their creator.

STORY

She had gone back to her home many months before and I no longer heard about her, but I used to visit her when she was still in the hospital and I am very confident that she is doing well at her home. She told that she was living alone all by herself in her apartment and it was indeed difficult for her because she had an amputation on the right side of her leg, but she was a strong woman, full of energy and determination. On my way to the office of the Chaplain, I was greeted with a smile by this woman, sitting in her wheeling chair. She asked if I still remembered her and I was stunned at first, because I couldn't really remember her exact name, so she introduced herself again. I looked at her and then I recalled our previous encounters. The stories and laughter we shared together, she even gave me religious books to read when she was still in the hospital. She told me that she was doing very well and she was at the hospital now for a follow up check up, but everything she was doing fine.

Looking at her she indeed had a smile all over her face and she looked good; she had gained weight but she really needed that. She was a woman of strong faith and she told me that she was never afraid to die, "We begin with Him and we end with Him," those were the words she left with me before her operation; but now she is really enjoying the gift of life and still has her contagious smile. She still held her rosary with her movable wheelchair and she was very happy we saw each other and shared a little of our stories and indeed she was right, that we begin and end with Christ. Our life is short we must try to be happy and enjoy it, for we have reason to enjoy it, our Savior is alive and brings joy to each and every one of us.

PRAYER
(PSALM 104: 1-6, 104: 31-33)
Bless the Lord, O my soul.
O Lord my God, you are very great.
You are clothed with honor and majesty,
Wrapped in the light as witha garment.
You stretch out the heavens like a tent,
You set the beams of your
Chambers on the waters,
You make the clouds your chariot,
You ride on the wings of the wind,
You make the winds your messengers,
Fire and flame your ministers.

You set the earth on its foundations,

So that it shall never be shaken.
You cover it with the deep as with a garment;
The water stood above the mountains.

May the glory of the Lord endure forever;
May the Lord rejoice in his works-
Who looks on the earth and it trembles,
Who touches the mountains and they smoke.
I will sing to the Lord as long as I live;
I will sing to my God while I have being.
Amen

TRUST

It is so rewarding at the end of the day when, we hear the Word of the master saying to us *"Well, done, good and trustworthy slave; you have been trustworthy in a few things I will put you in charge of many things so enter into the joy of the master."(*Mt. 25:1-30). Everything we see, everything we have, is entrusted to us by God. We try our best to care for, nourish and protect what He has given to us. God wants every one of us to be fruitful and produce good harvests; to produce a good harvest is to have good soil and good seed. I remember when I was young, my father after he retired from business decided to be a farmer; he planted rice and corn and it was very laborious at the very beginning. One way of planting rice, is to scatter the seeds to the surface of the soil that is free from any weeds and has a little water on the top of it. It can also be done on a seedbed first where the seed grows for few weeks until it becomes ready to transfer to the acre of ground ready for planting. My father used to wake up in the morning just to watch the seed grow and to watch the birds and pests that eat and attack it. He never missed a visit to his farm every day. Every time he went home, you can tell on his face what happened to his rice field. Pests and insects ate the leaves and the roots of the rice sometimes and he would tell us always what happened. There were times, he produced a good harvest, but there were times that he was so sad that his rice field did not produce a good one.

From the very beginning he was so watchful, right until the end. It is the love and devotion to his farm that brought the family to where we are now that was how he put his time and commitment to his family and in spite of the scorching sun and the time he invested waiting for the good harvest, he was not bothered at all. Indeed he was a hard working man, a good farmer, an excellent provider and a loving father to each one of us. He was just like St Joseph, a very simple quiet man and we love him. My father devoted his time to his family and to God and I do believe he is a faithful and trustworthy servant of God. I have seen a lot of people wasting their life, restless to accumulate material wealth. They invest their time and strength for personal glorification, and their unsatiable desire to have power, honor and glory for themselves, seems endless. Though God has given us everything we have materially, we know how to invest wealth not in things that pass and fade away but the kind of savings that would give us a place for eternity. In (Gen. 1; 26ff)God said: ***"Let us make humankind in our image according to our likeness; and let them have dominion over the fish of the sea and over the birds of the air and over the cattle and over all the wild animals of the earth and over every creeping thing that creeps upon the earth."***

God has given us dominion over all His creation but it also means we can abuse that privilege. It is given to us to enrich and do something to take care of the lives of future generations but it means that we don't look at what is best for the physical things, but for the spiritual growth that would last forever. True, that the loving God has given us life for us to nurture and to do the best we can in providing what we need, but what matters most at the end of the day, is the life that we had should be giving freely to the Giver, without hesitation, clean and undefiled. Praise is worthy to Him who has given a task for a certain calling or mission for a certain time. We shouldn't grieve so much when we leave this earth because, we do our best and we know that we are just passing travelers, and our permanent destination is to be with Him who sent us. I am very thankful as Chaplain in the hospital that most of the Catholic patients I administer to, have done their best and are leaving this place with so much peace and not holding on to anything. At the beginning of their journey, when their mother was there to see their first breath, so I was there as the person who would witness their last breath, as they bring back to God the breath they just borrowed. The life that we have is so precious yet fragile and we have to guard it, every moment of it, for we are accountable and responsible to present to the Giver at the end of our journey.

STORY

It was two thirty in the afternoon when the hospital called me but I missed that call and so after ten minutes they called me again. I was called to assist the social worker in explaining to the patient the things he needed to know. He was a Catholic, a very young man at the age of thirty nine years. He was working as a seaman on a ship that came from Japan and had stopped over at Nanaimo where they stayed for a little while. While there, he suffered a stroke and he was brought to the hospital where the findings of the medical expert was that he needed to have bypass surgery as soon as possible. This was his first time here in Victoria, and he was trying to figure things out; there were many things going through his head. He told me that it happened suddenly, and he did not know what to do. He signed many documents agreeing to treatment during his stay including the billing and the conditions that he might face regarding the operation. He had no immediate family members around and it seemed that he was just alone fighting for his life. His family was left in his country and his wife and two kids were also worried of his situation right now.

Most of the time, I just listened to his worries and apprehensions. His father was still coping with dialysis back home in Japan and he was worried about his finances. Well, it could happen to anyone; this is not his choice and I told him to take care of himself and to prepare mentally for the upcoming bypass surgery. In moments like this we have to trust God. We have to acknowledge the presence of the One who gives us life. He knows very much what we have been through and in this case, it's really beyond our power, we must leave every worry behind and think of the beautiful and wonderful things that God has given to us in this life.

In this case, faith really matters and this is when we can greatly use our understanding and our intimacy with God. This is when He shows His mercy and compassion in a closer way. If only we have that faith, we can really lighten the loads and burdens that we were facing. I knew at this moment in time that he needed to rest his mind and be patient and relax, the situation will not solve in just one night. It was then that he had to entrust not only his family back home in Japan to the hands of God but also the result of the upcoming surgery for him. He had to learn to trust to God as God entrusted to him the gift of life, and he in return must trust to God whatever happens along the journey. God knows very much what is good for us.

We prayed together and he received the Sacrament of Confession and Holy Communion, and I promised him I would visit him every time I did my rounds and would pray for the success of his surgery.

PRAYER
(PSALM 91: I -6, 91:14-16)
You who live in the shelter of the most High,
who abide in the shadow of the Almighty'
will say to the Lord, "My refuge and my fortress;
my God, in whom I trust."
For He delivers you from the snare of the fowler
and from the deadly pestilence;
He will recover you with His pinions,
and under His wings you will find refuge;
His faithfulness is a shield and buckler.

You will not fear the terror of the night,
or the arrow that flies by day,

or the pestilence that stalks in darkness
or the destruction that wastes at noonday.

Those who love me, I will deliver;
I will protect those who know my name.
when they call me, I will answer them;
I will be with them in trouble'
I will rescue them and honor them.
With long life I will satisfy them,
and show them my salvation.
Amen.

EUCHARIST

The most precious gift given to the priest is to become an "Alter Christus," to celebrate Mass and bring the real presence of Christ to the people. It is the definition of my priesthood, according to Second Vatican II (Presbyterorum Ordinis, No.4) which says: *"Eucharist is the center and the root of the whole priestly life." On the day before His death on the Cross, Christ instituted the Eucharist in the Upper Room. He offered Bread and Wine "…in His Sacred Hands"* (Roman Canon),and it became His Body and Blood offered in Sacrifice. Then He commanded His disciples to do this in memory of Him. Jesus is the life of the soul and He made himself available as food in the Sacrament of the Eucharist. Those who hunger and thirst will always be filled and satisfied. We heard the miracle story of the multiplication of bread in the Gospel of Luke (Lk. 9:16-17) which said: *"Jesus took the five loaves and the two fish, He looked up to heaven, and blessed and broke them, and He gave to His disciples to set before the crowd. And all ate and were filled."*

In the Gospel of John, (Jn. 6:48 -57) Jesus declared *"I am the bread of life, Your ancestors ate the manna in the wilderness, and they died. This is the bread that comes down from heaven, so that one may it of eat and not die. I am the living bread that came down from heaven. Whoever eats of this bread will live forever; and the bread that I will give for the life of the world is my flesh" The Jews then disputed among themselves, saying, "How can this man give us his flesh to eat"? so Jesus said to them, "Very truly, I tell you, unless you eat the flesh of the Son of Man and drink His blood, you have no life in you. Those who eat my flesh and drink my blood have eternal life, and I will raise them up on the last day; for my flesh is true food and my blood is true drink. Those who eat my flesh and drink my blood abide in me, and I in them, just as the living Father sent me, and I live because of the Father, so whoever eats me will live because of me. "* My life as a priest is not complete every day, without the celebration of the Eucharist. It is my joy to be with Christ every morning. It is my joy to reflect His words in my moment of silence. It is my joy to offer my life to him every day.

It is not the people at the altar during mass who complete the Eucharist, regardless of how many people participate. Christ completes the Eucharist. It is Christ who is present, who completes everything. The first letter of Paul to the Corinthians (1 Cor. 11:26) it says:

"...as often as you eat this bread and drink this cup you proclaim the Lord's death until He comes. " My own ministry at the hospital is really unique and challenging. When I worked in the Parish, usually I have a support group, I have good parishioners to deal with, but not in the hospital where everybody is in their bed. For me, it is only in the celebration of the Eucharist that I open my thoughts and feelings transparently to Jesus. He is my food, my strength and I ask him to take all away my heavy burdens and through the Holy Eucharist I renew my drooping spirit.

When a priest takes a day off, I hope and I pray that they still celebrate their daily mass. Such a holy celebration is very important in the life of the priest, before they begin or end the day. It is where we are renewed, strengthened, rooted and fed. While it is true in the life of a priest, it is also true to every individual Christian. **Catechism on Second Vat. Council on Document on the Sacred Liturgy** (No. 1324) says*: "It is the source and summit of the Christian life...for, in the Blessed Eucharist is contained the whole spiritual* *good of the church, Christ himself*. The paschal mystery of Christ is summarized in the Holy Eucharist but still can be ignored by many; some don't take it to heart. Some people are only nominal Christians who don't know the spiritual meaning of the celebration. In the Eucharist lies the very life of the church. It lies in the mystery of our faith, it lies in the joy of being a Christian, the joy of proclaiming that or faith is alive, for He is the risen. If only the whole congregation would know in a deepened sense that the Eucharist is the highest form of praise and thanksgiving, people would realize that going to mass everyday is not a waste of time but is fulfilling and satisfying. Perhaps we will see more people partaking of His Body and Blood at daily mass not just only on Sunday.

I still remember the story of the two disciples on the road to Emmaus. They were heartbroken, upset and hopeless and they thought everything was meaningless because Jesus was crucified and had died. They didn't really understand the teaching of Christ when He was with them, yet they prophesied that they knew the meaning of what the Prophet Isaiah in Chapter 53 said. Jesus was foretold as the suffering servant, but during the breaking of the bread, Jesus was made alive with them. This is also my experience in the hospital. People are lonely, frustrated and heartbroken because of their pain and sickness, but when they receive the Body of Christ, I can see the hope on their face, the joy within and the faith that they try to hang on to.

In the hospital though, sick people can't go to the church, but we have volunteers who bring Communion to them. They are committed and dedicated people who have been sent off by their pastors to bring the presence of Christ to patients in their beds. When we are not able to do so, because of physical incapability, God always provides a person to let us feel His presence and His love is still around, and I believe that the volunteers who bring them the Body of Christ are sent by God in a very concrete way, letting them know that God is around and feeding them through these untiring workers in His vineyard.

STORY

Seldom had I heard the voice of this woman; she spoke very little and I did not really know where she lived or her family background, but I knew that besides the doctor and nurses, there were some good people who visited her from time to time. I saw pots of beautiful flowers around every now and then and cards wishing for her immediate recovery that the nurses put on her wall. She was a woman of few words, mysterious. Every time I made my visit, I always wore a hospital gown and gloves because she was situated in the isolation room and the first time I met her she was listening to music; she had her own radio besides her bed and she was always sitting in the rocking chair looking out of the window, probably to see the birds flying freely outside or to see the sun shining freely and brightening up the day.

She seldom had a smile on her face but when I looked at her she always told me "I want Communion." Those were the clear words I always heard from her. She always had a time for prayer. and every time we started our prayer, she would tell me to turn off the radio for she could not reach by her herself, she was frail and tired. We prayed together and I could see she was a woman of great faith. We prayed the Apostle's Creed, the Our Father, the Hail Mary and Glory Be, and I was surprised that she still remembered them off by heart. It was the Eucharist which was the precious gift I gave her every time I made my rounds and she was always waiting for that. She was always waiting for my coming and she knew very well that every time she saw me coming she was going to receive the Body of Christ. She was indeed, the silent daughter of God, longing to see God face to face someday, somehow, the Body of Christ that I brought to her every day, not only gave her spiritual nourishment but also gave her the presence of Christ which is always available, faithful to the very end. I hope and

I pray she will see the presence of His son, the Savior soon, but not yet.

PRAYER
(PSALM 118: 1-4-28-29)
O give thanks to the Lord, for He is good;
His steadfast love endures forever!
Let Israel say,
"His love endures forever."
Let the house of Aaron say,
"His love endures forever."
Let those who fear the Lord say
"His love endures forever."

You are my God, and I will give thanks to you;
And you are my God, I will extol you.
O give thanks to the Lord for he is good, for his love endures forever.
Amen.

CROSS

"Lord, by your Holy Cross, you have redeemed the world." We pray this simple prayer when we make the Stations of the Cross during Lent; it is indeed a very simple phrase that really captures the true meaning of the cross. Before and after every prayer, at every spiritual ritual, when passing the church, or sometimes when we feel in danger, or are feeling fear, as a Catholic we give ourselves the sign of the cross; that reminds us of our faith. This is the same cross we see in every Catholic house, rectories of parishes, seminary formation houses and every convent, in the nun's rooms and chapels. In every Catholic school they usually have bigger crosses visible to the students

It is interesting to know that we have a similarity of doing things with Jews; Jesus did this practice for he was a Jew. The single sentence we find in the book of Deuteronomy (6:4) says:

"Hear, O Israel, the Lord is our God, the Lord alone." This is the real creed of the Jewish people and it is called the Shema. It is a single sentence that the Jews in the synagogue always use to start their service by reciting, until now. It is their creed that declares that their God is the only God. The Shema is contained in a little box, called the Mezuzah and they affix this on every door of their house, to remind them of God as they leave the house and as they come back.

In (Matthew 23:5) it says: *"They do all their deeds to be seen by others; for they make their phylacteries broad and their fringes long."* The word phylacteries refers to the little boxes which the scribes and Pharisees and devout Jews wore on their foreheads and on their wrists when they were at service in the synagogue. Like the

Catholics, we start and end our prayer by making on ourselves the sign of the cross, the Jewish people recite the Shema when they begin their service.

I guess, the point of comparing the two rituals is because, Jesus was a Jew, at the same time He is the founder of the new people of God, and Christianity. But I guess, I have to stop here, comparing the ritual of Catholic Christians and Jewish people. I want to dwell the more on the deeper meaning of the cross as a Christian where I can relate more on my own experiences and the people who are sick. In Matthew (16:24-25) states: ***"Then Jesus told His disciples, if any want to become my followers, let them deny themselves and take up their cross and follow me."*** For some people the cross is too heavy and hard to carry and sometimes if you don't know the spiritual meaning of your cross, you could easily become upset and frustrated in life.

An eighty three year old Catholic woman was diagnosed with cancer and I was called to the hospital at eight in the morning because she wanted to pour out her emotions after finding out that she had a cancer. She was so lonely and in terrible pain and she knew that she was not young or ready to meet the husband who died five years before, but for this moment, she wanted to free herself from any pains in her body and she wanted mainly to ease the pain in her stomach. We prayed together and at the very end of our prayer she would interrupt and say "If this is the way she can help carry the cross of Christ, so be it." She is a woman of great faith, I met her nephew and daughter and they highly spoke of the spiritual values of this woman, indeed, every time I visited her, she was so delighted and was longing to receive the Body of Christ.

I have seen a lot of people who find carrying their cross so heavy especially those people who don't recognize the presence of God in their lives; they are the ones who easily get upset and frustrated. They are the ones who rely on their human strength and they are the ones who never know that in this moment of difficulties, the value of prayer is very important. I have had my own share of carrying the cross, when my youngest brother died and I was in the seminary. I still remember I really didn't know what to do. I must admit I was so close to him and I loved him, he was my favorite brother and I was in terrible despair and lost. It seemed that part of my inner body also died and I was about to give up my calling. I was broken hearted and I didn't really know how to step forward and focus on my studies in the seminary so I left for a little while because I couldn't focus myself on the formation and my community life. That, was thirteen years ago but still the memory of loss is still there.

Our life as a Christian is to carry the cross every day. We are living in a world where what the world offers to us is contrary to our Christian values, and we are challenged in how to live out the calling of a true disciple of Christ. For those who don't believe in Jesus; for them the cross is strange and a kind of punishment or bad luck. But for us as Catholic Christians this s the way it is. We must remember, Jesus never said to us, "If you want to be my follower you will be free of sorrow and you will become rich and famous." If we surrender our self to the grace of God everything will have a direction, everything will have a beautiful meaning. We don't end on the cross we have but we connect our cross to the cross of Christ. By His cross He was gloried, by that cross, He saved us. We have to embrace our cross with a humble heart, and rely on the grace of God to help us carry it. We hear so many priests telling us in their homilies that God will not give us a cross that is so heavy that we cannot bear or carry. He is always there to help us to carry it. What He needs from us is the humility to accept, to love and to embrace that cross. The cross purifies us and makes us closer to Him and He is inviting us to call on His name. He will not remove the cross that we have, but perhaps but He will accompany us in our journey.

When we find the spiritual meaning of the cross, tat cross will turn into joy and privilege for letting us experience the meaning of the cross in our life. The cross is our identity as a Catholic Christian; every time you see a person making the sign of the cross, you know that he/she is a Catholic, and that we are very grateful because we are not ashamed of telling the people that this is a gift, this is our faith and we find joy in doing it because we see the whole meaning of what to be a Catholic Christian means, the joy of finding the smiling face of Christ in the midst of heavy burdens and the heavy cross we carry every day. We forget the hardship, but we always feel the joy because in Christ He always turns our sorrow into joy, our cross into glory. The cross stands for our faith.

STORY

On my rounds at the hospital, I met this man, he looked young for his age and he wanted to talk to me in the corridor, but the first time we met, I was rushing to see a dying person and her family in another room. I know he wanted to talk to me that time, but it did not happen. The following day, I saw a new name on the list and it said that he wanted to see a priest, so I went along to his room. I found him talking with this young boy whom I was told was his son from Alberta who was here to visit his dad. This man worked in Mexico for more than five years and he loved to be There, his business was doing so well in Mexico and he wanted to find a good woman after his wife had died four years ago. He wanted to start a new family there, but he had to see his family doctor in Mexico because he felt sick all the time, was dizzy and had lost his appetite and it was something that bothered him so much. He decided to visit his home here in Victoria and while here, he went to the hospital for a check-up and he found out that he had terminal leukemia, cancer of the blood. The first time I met him, he told me about his life in Mexico; his happy moments and dreams for his retirement, but he was not prepared at all, for everything happened very quickly. I listened to him and his wonderful experiences in Mexico then I gave him Communion and then the Sacrament of the Sick.

A few visits later, he told me that he was okay and ready to go home. After a month I saw him again at the hospital, for the second time and this time I could hardly recognize him. He was thin and frail and he had lost the smile on his face; it seemed that he was facing a tremendous blow in his life. The third time, (and this was not an easy one), the immediate family members and friends were there. He was delirious and his condition was really going downhill so much so that he had been given just twenty four hours to live. I introduced myself to him and to his one daughter who was present; the other three were still expected to come at any moment. I saw his fear and loneliness and I thought that he was too young to die, but the daughter told me that it was not too young, for in their family sixty five years old was good enough. They knew not to plan their retirement years for it will not happen because they inherited the genes and blood that runs in their families.

We prayed together and a lot of friends came, starting from just a few until I saw there was not enough room for us all inside. I explained to them the meaning of the cross of Christ and that suffering and pain is part of human existence, but we know that we are all caretakers of this life and soon the One who gives this life will take it away from us, for we are not the owner. His will be done always, not our will. The cross looks painful and humiliating but in that same disgrace, the resurrection comes and new life begins. I believe that for this man, undergoing such a tremendous challenge and facing death, the only remedy is to see the cross of Christ and connect it to the cross that we have, so that Jesus will take what we have and make it His own. Before I leave, all of us prayed together for the healing of this man, if not of his physical aspect, but for his spiritual healing and purification.

May God grant him peace and forgiveness and recognize him as one of his sheep.

PRAYER
(PSALM 23: 1-6)
The Lord is my shepherd, I shall not want.
He makes me lie down in green pastures;
He leads me beside still waters;
He restores my soul.
He leads me in the right paths
For His name's sake.

Even though I walk through the darkest valley,
I fear no evil;
For you are with me;
Your rod and your staff-
They comfort me.

You prepared a table for me
in the presence of my enemies,
You anoint my head with oil;
My cups overflows.

Surely goodness and mercy shall follow me
all the days of my life,
and I shall dwell in the house of the Lord
My whole life long.
Amen.

HEALING

We read so many stories of miracles in the Holy Bible. We read and we were touched by the different healings of Jesus. He healed the lame, the crippled, the blind, the deaf, the paralyzed, lepers, mutes, women with hemorrhages, those who had fevers, and even gave life back to those who had lost their battle against their sickness. When we read the miracle of healing, it seemed that we are also healed not only physically but spiritually. In the Gospel of Matthew(Mt. 8: 5-10) it says: *"When He entered Capernaum, a centurion came to Him, appealing toHim and saying "Lord my servant is lying at home paralyzed, in terrible distress. And He said to him, "I will come and cure him." The centurion answered, "Lord, I am not worthy to have you under my roof; but only speak the word and my servant will be healed. For I also am a man under authority, with soldiers under me; and I say to one, 'Go' and he goes and to another,' Come' and he comes and to my slave, 'Do this' and the slave does it. When Jesus heard him, He was amazed and said to those following Him, "Truly I tell you, in no one in Israel have I found such faith."* These humble words of the centurion before Jesus became our words before we receive His body during Communion. We also confess these words. *"Lord I am not worthy to receive you but only say the word and I will be healed."*

So simple, so humbling yet powerful.

The dialogue of the centurion is not about the cure or about his slave but it is all about the Healer, about Jesus. His very encounter with Jesus gave him affirmation of his strong faith though he was a Roman soldier. His very encounter with Jesus paved the way to those believers of Christ regardless of our human origin. In the Gospel of Luke (Lk. 17:11-19) it tells that Jesus cleanses the ten lepers. These ten lepers approached Jesus for a cure and they were healed. Nine left but the one who was a Samaritan went back to thank Jesus. The nine were restored physically in their relationship with people and with their families but the one who gave thanks to Jesus not only healed both physically and spiritually but developed a deeper intimacy with Jesus. His very encounter is a testimony of his renewed faith.

Each healing is a personal witnessing to the power of Christ and that's why wherever He went, the people followed Him for healing. I do believe that physical sickness is just peripheral and that the pain goes deeper, meaning that it is also the spiritual sickness that needs to be cured.

This is what I found in those who had their faith. It is really very easy for them to accept their suffering and their illness because they know that sickness can destroy the body but not the spirit. They know it can only solidify and sanctify the soul because of the pain and suffering that the sick person endures to the end.

The presence of the priest as an instrument of God's healing power that needs not to be ignored and it really helps those who need healing internally. In the Gospel of John (Jn. 20:19-23) it states: *"Now when it was late that same day, the first of the week, and the doors were shut where the disciples were gathered together for fear of the Jews, Jesus came and stood in their midst, and said to them: "Peace be with you." And when He said this, He showed him His hands and His side. The disciples therefore were glad, when they saw the Lord. He said therefore to them again: "Peace be with you. As the Father hath sent me, I also send you." When He had said this, He breathed on them; and He said to them: "Receive you the Holy Spirit. Whose sins you shall forgive, they are forgiven them; and whose sins you shall retain they are retained.*" Christ uses His priests as His instruments of healing, especially in the Sacrament of Confession. It is an experience of liberation from the slavery of sins; we become free and Jesus rejoices to forgive and heal us. As a Chaplain in the hospital I have witnessed countless healings, some of them so simple and it is reasonable to cure that kind of sickness but some of them I called miracles, when even the doctors and nurses try to explain and can't find scientific reasons for the cure. They themselves can't find the answer and neither did their books or their schools mention it either.

Healing is what everybody is looking for in the hospital; healing from the physical sickness that cripples their day to day existence, bothers their plans and ruins the whole system of living. Physical healing is only peripheral and easy to heal, but there is a deeper kind of woundedness that needs healing too, and that is the inner and spiritual healing. People nowadays are timid and reserved to open up their true feelings and situations, they will cover up their shortcomings and mistakes rather than talk openly, air their sentiment and be heard. I have seen people who have been healed after their stay in the hospital, not only of their physical wounds but mostly the spiritual aspect of their lives. Life is so short that the second time around, they will treasure their life in every moment of the day. And faith helps us to grow as a person and, we know that it happens for a reason.

STORY

My encounter with this woman was different for many reasons. Before I met her, she phoned me many times because she wanted to have Confession in the middle of the night and I explain to her about the gift of the Sacrament and to not talk over the phone so as to preserve the sanctity of this rite. Every minute, she used the private telephone at the hospital to talk to me. Since I was new to this ministry, I didn't really know what kind of sickness she had as she sounded well and had many stories to tell. After a week I found out where exactly she was; she was in this building which catered for those people who suffer from depression and severe addiction. When I found her, she told me why she ended up in this building for twenty years of her life. She told me that she was like a bird without wings that can't easily survive outside because there is a certain limit to the time allowed for a stay outside.

She told me her story, how she was married twenty years ago, with a Catholic wedding. She has a son who is twenty three years old right now and she told me that he is doing well, has a good job; is still single and used to visit her in this building. She was proud of her son; she always mentioned that to me. She got depressed when the husband filed for a divorce from her and this was the downfall of her life. Everything changed and she was not able to cope with the demands of married life, especially with regard to the man she loved so much and then lost. She told me the main reason why she was divorced by her husband; she had made a great mistake and her husband did not give her another chance. She was angry at herself and even until now she can't forget the past. Along the way, she hooked up with bad influences involving alcohol and smoking that even until now she is still fighting to get rid of. She told me that her life was monotonous, lifeless, and was nothing worth holding on to. She was confined to that building for more than twenty years and longs for when she will be able to be free.

Every time I visited her, she told me that the doctor had been to see her and she hoped everything would be fine for her to be released within a year, so she could start another life and find new job to start. When she will be free I don't know, only time can tell, but in our prayers, we always prayed for her. I prayed for the best. I wanted to see her free and start over all again and I want to see her to be able to stand up and continue to move forward. Life for some is cruel and she was one of those who saw life as difficult. I believe she deserved healing for both her body and soul and she needed to forget about the past and look for the brighter side that life may bring. I want to see her fulfilling her dreams and to be able to find meaning in her existence. She is still very young at the age of forty three and she is still very connected with her experience in the church; she still believed the presence of Jesus in our midst and she was still longing to receive the Body of Christ every time I made my visit. Although it seemed that her life was already at a dead end, I am hoping against hope that healing will come upon her one day. Only her own prayer and discipline can bring healing to the deep seated wounds that haunt her every now and then my prayer goes out to her, for she deserves the beauty of God's gift of life and the wonder of God's creation.

PRAYER
(PSALM 41: 1-4)
Happy are those who consider the poor;
The Lord delivers them in the day of trouble.
The Lord protects them and keeps them alive;
They are called happy in the land.
You do not give them up to the will of their enemies.
The Lord sustains them on their sickbed;
In their illness you heal all their infirmities.
As for me I said, O Lord, be gracious to me;
Heal me, for I have sinned against you.
Amen.

REPENTANCE

In the Gospel of Mark (Mk. 1:3-4) it says: *"...hear the voice of one crying out in the wilderness "Prepare the way of the Lord make His path straight." John the baptizer appeared in the wilderness, proclaiming a baptism of repentance for the forgiveness of sins. "*I have been a priest for only seven years, still relatively young in my ministry, but I am fortunate enough to experience the many facets of my calling. I was an Associate, an Administrator and now a hospital Chaplain; this I love and I am devoted to my ministry. It is a gift, it is a privilege, it is chosen by the hands of God and I have that tremendous joy of serving Him through His people.

For seven years of ministry, I have encountered a repentant who has confessed to me. "Father," he said, "I don't know where to start, but I was away from the church for forty two years, and since then, I have never been to Confession. Help me Father, I don't know what to do, I do not know where to start." He said, "I just want to bring myself back to church because for many years I have drifted away; I lost my track, have a lot of sins and mistakes and I hurt many people," I was surprised he was crying, and he was so honest to tell me all the stories in his life that need to be forgiven. I told him that, the Sacrament of Confession is the sacrament where we experience the loving embrace of God, his overflowing of mercy and compassion. We talked for almost an hour but at the end I saw his face smiling and he was ready to take a chance for a new life, a new hope, a new beginning for the remaining of his life and his family.

We are all wounded, lost and broken, indeed we are, but if we surrender ourselves to Him and allow ourselves to open our heart for His blessing and grace He is really happy to take care of us. But we have to repent first, we have to be honest and sincere that we can move on and not sin anymore. If there is a place for ninety nine who did not lose their way, there is always a time for searching, and a special place for the one who did go astray. Like the story of the prodigal son and the lavish love of the father who every moment of his life, every minute of the day, was standing at the door, looking somewhere at the end of sunset hopeful that someday his prodigal son will return to his embrace. He was full of longing and that is the image I have for the sinners like us who want to humble themselves to stand naked in the eyes of God.

The Sacrament of Confession has a lifetime benefit that no matter how broke you are in life, financially or spiritually and regardless of your status and role in society, I assure you, you will receive the same benefits from God. It is a life time guarantee that you can carry over until the next life with so many interests and benefits. I was called early in the morning at around two am, to give the last rite for a dying man. I was surprised that the whole family was there because they came from different provinces of Canada. They wanted to see their dad, fighting for his last breath. I was surprised that one of the daughters asked for Confession after I had given my prayer and the Sacrament of the Sick to the dying father. She said, "At this moment, I surrender him to the Lord. He was sick for seven years and I really pitied him. He was in and out of the hospital, his body deteriorated and every time I saw him I couldn't help him. I can't bring him to sustain his life again, I just don't know, but I do believe in the power of God, He can do what would be the best for our dad and also for each one of us, for my mom and the rest of the family." She asked if she could have the Sacrament of Confession, because it may be the only way that she can help him during this crucial moment. I said to her, "Well, we have no place here, we will have to go outside in the corridor at the bench." and that was where I heard her confession, Then she said, "Stay here Father and just wait." I waited and their mom, four sisters and two brothers came to me for the Sacrament of Confession. It was one of the most fruitful ministries I ever carried out in the hospital. They were not able to save the life of their father but I do believe, their father found a life where is there no death anymore, no hospital gadgets attached to the body, no needles, no medicine. A place where everybody wants to be peaceful and live in lasting happiness; living with the saints and angels and all the biblical characters whom we read about. We meet them in person and we meet our Creator face to face with so much awe and jubilation.

Repentance is a beautiful gift given by Jesus in the church. It is a sacrament that makes us spoiled sons and daughters and it is given every time we have done wrong, every time we need his embrace and comforting words. The Sacrament of Repentance is the right medicine to cure and heal our ailing spirit. Nowadays, it is sad to say, few Catholics really appreciate and want to avail of this precious gift. St. John Vianney spent more than sixteen hours in the confessional box, just to listen and heal the brokenness of people all over the world, and I hope and pray that conversion happens along the way. People nowadays have become more self-centered and proud that they think they don't need the sacrament, they don't need to go for confession, and it has really drastically changed them, it seems they don't really know about this sacrament.

Catholics struggle to live out the meaning of this sacrament because they are living around the other denominations who don't believe in the Sacrament of Confession, but I hope and I pray that the church will continue to hold on to this beautiful sacrament, where we can experience the loving presence of the Father embracing his prodigal son and daughter after a long journey of loss and shame.

Nothing changes after our return home except that this time, we can feel the loving mercy of the Father and His pouring out of time and care for the wounded traveler becoming closer and very intimate.

STORY

I was called to give the Sacrament of the Sick to a person. His wife called me and requested that I visit him and she told me the background history of her husband; that for more than ten years he had walked away from the church and since then he had never returned. He is now confined to the hospital at eighty eight years old and was diagnosed with cancer but still was not planning to return to the church. The first time I saw him he told me about his anger and frustration with the church that he used to serve. He was one of the pillars of their parish, very active in the church activities but was so scandalized one time that he turned his back on the church he used to love. I sat there at his bedside for an hour, just to listen to what he was saying. He vented his anger and aired his sentiments and feelings to me but in spite of what he experienced in the church, he never changed religion. Most of the time I just listened to what he said but in the back of my mind I prayed for him to have a change of heart along the way. The fact that he called a priest is an indication that he was open for reconciliation and peace. At the end of our meeting I saw his teary eyes and his emotion that he too greatly missed his life in the church. He missed the mass, the sacraments and his friends who were churchgoers.

I prayed for him and I always continue my prayer for him. His return would always be a good sign that the Catholic Church is not holding any grudges toward anyone and it is flowing with mercy and compassion for those who seek forgiveness. I hope that before it's too late, this patient would experience the loving kindness and forgiveness of the church and see that it is the best gift he could offer to himself, to God and his people, especially his wife who prayed for him. Forgiveness is a beautiful gift from God and although it is like standing naked in front of God telling our shameful and mistakes, our shortcomings and sins, at the end it is how we also experience the embrace of the Heavenly Father who is always waiting for our return, like the story of the prodigal son. It renews our ailing and drooping soul. I never heard of him anymore, but my constant prayer for him is always there and I hope for the best, that one day he would return and enjoy the gift and blessing that he missed so much. I pray that at the end of the journey, before he closed his eyes, he would see the hands of Christ trying to comfort him and bless him and bring him peace and Joy. Yes, I do pray for him.

PRAYER
(PSALM 32: 1-2; 5-7;11)
Happy are those whose transgression is forgiven,
whose sin is covered.
Happy are those to whom
the Lord imputes no iniquity,
and in spirit there is no deceit.

Then I acknowledged my sin to you,
and did not hide my iniquity;
I said "I will confess my transgressions
To the Lord,"
And you forgave the guilt of my sin.

Therefore let all who are faithful
Offer prayer to you;
At a time of distress, the rush of mighty waters
Shall not reach them.
You are a hiding place for me;
You preserve me from trouble;
You surround me with glad and deliverance.

Be glad in the Lord and rejoice,
O righteous,
And shout for joy, all you
Upright in heart.
Amen.

1 (ST PAUL & THE CHAPLAIN)

In the letter of Paul to the Galatians (Gal. 2: 20) it says: *"...and it is no longer I who live, but it is Christ who lives in me And the life I now live in the flesh I live by faith in the Son of God."* As I tried to start my reflection on the Word, I was recalling the words of St. Paul when all of a sudden I found them and remembered that these beautiful words set the tone for all servants working in the Lord's vineyard; that is proclaiming the word of God, and doing His mission. It is not 'I' in the center of interest but God himself. Preaching is self emptying and we empty our self interest and self glorification so that the true meaning of the Word of God will communicate so well to the heart and mind of the people. I must admit, some priests, some lay persons and some people who are evangelizers and pastors are gifted in eloquent public speaking; they were born with honey on their lips; it is a gift, a gift that can attract people to listen to what they are proclaiming. It is a gift because I know, not all people can do such powerful preaching in public, and I have seen a lot. But again, if we use it for the greater glory of God we are very grateful for sharing the gift, but if we do it for self serving purposes, for our self gratification, that would be a very misleading example.

Some priests and some lay evangelizers we see on TV are very popular because they have the power of sending the message of the gospel to the people. They can really relate to the life of the listeners and people flock to listen to their preaching and again, if it is done with good intention, then so be it. St. Paul emptied himself to become the immortal preacher of the Gentiles and for the whole church. He emptied himself so that the Mission of Christ would be carried out and realized. He did not speak in and of himself but always in the name Christ and Christ was the center of his preaching. I know working for the sick at the hospital is more humbling in a way; any nurses, doctors, and family members can call me to visit the patient. I know very much that in serving them, regardless of life, is a way of doing the mission of Christ in a very simple way; when He was on earth, He was a healer. The people did not come only because he was an excellent preacher but because he was also a healer. He healed so many sick people and all the four gospels of the four evangelists have all the accounts of the healing miracles done by Jesus. And those people who were privileged to see him were healed not only of their physical illness but also the spiritual.

I act in the name of Christ and I have nothing to be proud of myself because everything I do comes from the gift of my priesthood, I perform my ministry in His name. St Paul in his letter to the Galatians(Gal 5: 14) says: *"...may I never boast of anything except the cross of our Lord Jesus Christ by which the world has been crucified to me, and I to the world."* Yes, indeed like St Paul we have nothing to be proud of with other people, the gifts that we have are given to us for a purpose, to bring the Good News of salvation and always, Christ is the center of our actions. Even Jesus Himself when He was performing miracles never forgot to mention His Father, to thank Him and acknowledge Him, and he is doing this so that His Father will be known and revealed to the people. The Gospel of John (Jn.11:40-44) states: *"Jesus told her, "Did I not tell you that if you believed, you will see the glory of God?" So they took away the stone. And Jesus looked upward and said, "Father, I thank you for having heard me. I knew that you always hear me, but I have said this for the sake of the crowd standing here, so that they may believe that you sent me."*

Jesus and the Father are one; they love each other, they have a very intimate relationship with each other. Before coming here in the world Jesus was with the Father, that's why all the preaching of Jesus was about loving, forgiving and glorifying His Father.

In the Gospel of John (Jn. 12:27-28) it says: *"Father, glorify your name." Then the voice came from heaven, "I have glorified it, and I glorified them again."* When we preach, and when we give the homily, the center of our story is no other than our encounter with Jesus who sent us to proclaim the Good News by virtue of our ordination. We do not speak of ourselves but it is all about Christ, we have a personal intimate relationship with Christ and we are one with Him. We were taught all this theological formation in the seminary where we were formed to imitate Him, and although imperfect, we tried, in our preaching, not to become self centered that people might believe not in us but the One who called us and sent us as His envoy to the world. Again the Gospel of John (Jn. 12: 44-45*)* states: *"...then Jesus cried aloud: "Whoever believes in me believes not in me but Him who sent m. and whoever sees me sees Him who sent me."*

The encounters we have with Jesus would inspire the life of others to know the Lord in a very personal way. In fact he calls us by name during our Baptism, to establish a real personal friendship with Him. Sometimes, I have reason to travel early in the middle of the night and at the wee hours of the morning to bring the Body of Christ to the sick and like St. Paul, in his personal encounter with Jesus on his way to Damascus, it showed him the urgency to travel to preach and bring the Good News of salvation to the pagan nations. It is really a joy serving in the name of Christ. I act on my personal friendship with Jesus and I believe I became a priest for no other reason than to be sent out because I had developed and intimate friendship with Him.

There is an inner joy when I feel that I have brought my friendship with Jesus to the patient and family members and they feel at peace and contented.

The letter of Paul to the first Corinthians (1 Cor. 15: 8-11) says: *"But by the grace of God. But by the grace of God I am what I am, and His grace toward me has not been in vain. On the contrary, I worked harder than any of them—though it was not I, but the grace of God that is with me. Whether then it was I or they, so we proclaim and so you have come to believe."*

I would like to give an expression of gratitude to my fellow Chaplains who work at the hospital, thanks for their unselfish service and their joy in fulfilling their calling as servants of the Lord especially those who are able and not sick. The Chaplains of the hospital that I work with indeed are true servants of God; friendly and ever loving and caring. They are really called to this special ministry for the sick. I was inspired the first time I met this one particular Chaplain; he was so eager to help me and give me directions. He told me a little bit of his experience in the hospital like the importance of privacy and confidentiality and he told me also a little bit of his family back ground and the joy of his service at the end of the day. I can't find the right words to describe his energy, his gift of presence, his smile to all the people, patients and personnel working at the hospital. He is a good man and through his presence he has broken the line of boundaries among different religions, he is there not only for his own religion but for all. His gift of presence is a gift to everybody and he is always there with a comforting word and kindness to all the sick. I reflect on that when we are doing our ministry, it is Christ who acts in us and it is the compassionate and loving Christ that is living in us. Yes, serving the sick we Chaplains never take on what is comfortable to us, it is always for the love and care of the sick that we think and serve first; the presence of Christ must be seen in our actions and words.

Often I had heard good things about the two Chaplains, mostly from the Catholic patients who spoke in high regard and respect about them. Indeed, they serve not only for themselves but always in the name of Christ. We always set aside our personal gratification so that the mercy and love of God will be seen through our presence. Yes, indeed it is no longer us, or I that lives but Christ that lives in us and I, with my fellow Chaplains, am glad to share this joy with the sick people we love at the hospital. That the loving mercy of Jesus will be seen and revealed through us, is who we are, humble 'Alter Christus' of Jesus. Hospital Chaplain's love to serve and our service will never end, as the love of Christ for the sick never ends.

PRAYER
(PSALM 63: 1-4)
O God you are my God, I seek you,
my souls thirst for you;
My flesh faints for you,
as in dry and weary land
Where is no water.
So I have looked upon you
in the sanctuary,
Beholding your power and glory.
Because your steadfast love
is better than life,
my lips will praise you.
So I will bless you as long as I live;
I will lift up my hands and call on your name.
Amen.

SPIRIT

Most of the people to whom I gave the last rite, that is the Sacrament of the Sick, they were people who were about to die and sadly to say, usually the family members call the priest at the last minute when a person can't talk and can't receive the Body of Christ. The patient can't decide by herself/himself what to do although when look on the silent face of the dying patients they are filled with sorrow and sadness that the most precious gift, the Body of Christ, they can't even have in this last and important moment on earth. But on the other hand, their sadness after a little while, will turn into joy when their heart is set to see their God face to face and no longer in a dim mirror.

Most of us fall many times and we drift away from His 'track' we go in a different direction that leads to nowhere. People may lose sight of Christ for a certain time or even the whole period of their journey, but at the very end they choose to encounter Him like the repentant thief before he died asked Jesus to welcome him into his paradise. And then at that moment, death is transformed into life, a new life with Christ; it is no longer a sad ending but a glorified ending.

The letter of Paul to the Romans (Rm. 8: 17) tells us: *"...for those who live according to the flesh set their minds on the things of the flesh, but those who live according to the Spirit set their minds on the things of the Spirit. To set their mind on the flesh is death, but to set the mind on the Spirit is life and peace. For this reason the mind that is set on the flesh is hostile to God; it does not submit to God's law—indeed it cannot and those who are in the flesh cannot please God."* But we are not in the flesh we are in the Spirit of God through the indwelling of the Holy Spirit during the Sacrament of Baptism and strengthened when we receive the gifts of the Spirit during the Sacrament of Confirmation. We will die yes, our body will return unto dust because of sin but our spirit will live because of righteousness. *"We are all sons and daughters of God, heirs of His kingdom and do not let your heart be troubled, don't be sad."* (Rm. 8:18).

St Paul says: *"I consider that the sufferings of this present time are not worth comparing with the glory about to be revealed to us."* When Jesus Christ died His disciples were plunged into sadness and despair too but when Jesus resurrected and ascended to the right hand of the Father He sent the Holy Spirit, and then the sorrow and sadness of the disciples turned into joy. In John (14: 25-27) it says: *"I have said these things to you while I am still with you. But the advocate, the Holy Spirit, whom the Father will send in my name, will teach you everything and remind you of all that I have said to you. Peace I leave with you; my peace I give to you. I do not give to you as the world gives. Do not let your hearts be troubled, and do not let them be afraid."* The disciples, though they were broken hearted when Jesus left, were comforted and filled with fire in their hearts to do their mission. They traveled to all different parts of the world and they shed their blood to pay the price for proclaiming the Good News but they were able to shine while on their mission and did what Jesus commanded them to do. Do not be afraid.

The apostles felt the presence of the Holy Spirit and that they were not alone. The Holy Spirit strengthened them and made them the true and faithful disciples of Christ. In the letter of St Paul (Gal 5: 22-23), he says: *"...by contrast, the fruit of the spirit is love, joy, peace, patience, kindness, generosity, faithfulness, gentleness, and self control.* I know that when a person dies, his body will return to dust, for we are dust and unto dust we shall return, but our spirit is alive and will never die waiting for the coming of our Savior. We have to turn our misery and sorrow to the death of Christ, as in His death He found new life. He vindicated death and it no longer has power over Him and that is what Jesus is telling and challenging us about. In the letter of Paul to the Galatians (Gal. 6: 8), he says: *"If you sow to your flesh, you will reap corruption from the flesh; but if you sow to the spirit, you will reap eternal life from the Spirit."* I am very thankful for all the patients that I have administered to in the hospital although most of them I met only in their dying moments but regardless of what their life had been in the past, at the very end of their life I saw their turning point. They chose life rather than death and in doing so, they chose Christ, their hearts longing to see Him face to face.

STORY

I was called to the hospital to give the last rite to an eighty five year old man. He couldn't talk and I couldn't understand most of his gestures but I was surprised, because the first time he saw me, he recognized me as a priest. With his weary hands he tried to make the sign of the cross on his body and when he looked at me, I saw the tears that kept coming from his half closed eyes. I was moved with pity and then suddenly the nurses and the daughter and his sister told me to leave for a little while as they were fixing the bed but he was fixing his face on me.

After few minutes, I asked his daughter and sister to leave us for a little while, because I had asked him if he wanted me to hear his confession. Though I couldn't hear him that much or understand what he was saying I gave him absolution because of his willingness to ask forgiveness and ask for this sacrament. Thank God that at that moment he also received the Sacrament of the Sick and the Body of Christ which he surely missed when he was still strong.

Afterwards, I invited the daughter and the sister to come in and they told me the story of this person when he was still young and able to serve his church. He grew up as an altar server and married in a Catholic wedding, but after that he was too busy dealing with his business that he drifted away from the church service. His daughter told me that he was a good father, a faithful husband and a good provider to his family, also his wife had died five years before and now he was going to meet her. She said to me "I just want to let you know Father that this really is the wish of my father, to have confession with the priest and to receive the Sacrament of the Sick and to receive His body. Thank you for coming in." We sang the Salve Regina when I left and I am very happy that at the end of his earthly journey he was able to meet the forgiving and loving Jesus in the presence of the priest.

I am very happy that though he drifted away from spiritual values in his earthly life, what mattered to him at the end, which was the concern of his spirit; the spirit that was revealed to him then. It was more important than those earthly things that he spent too much time with. What mattered most at the very end was that his spirit longed to see his Creator, the Giver of life, the meaning of all our lives, who is Jesus himself.

PRAYER
(PSALM 77: 1-3, 11-15)
I cry aloud to God,
aloud to God, that He may hear me.
In the day of my trouble I seek the Lord;
In the day of my hand is stretched out
without wearying;
My soul refuses to be comforted.
I think of God and I moan;
I meditate and my spirit faints.

I will call to mind the deeds of the Lord;
I will remember your wonders of old.

I will meditate on all your work,
And muse on your mighty deeds.
Your way, O God is Holy.
What God is so great with our God
You are the God who works wonders;
with your strong arms
You redeemed your people,
The descendants of Jacob and Joseph.
Amen.

THANKSGIVING

It is interesting to know that in most of the writings of St Paul, he started with salutation followed by giving thanks and praise to God. This is also the very intention of writing this book, to bring me back to God, to praise and glorify His name forever, though St Paul always put his gratitude at the very beginning and I use it at the very end of this book. I like St Paul, that's why I was able to read and review all his writings and compare with what I have learned in my theology year in the seminary and in the new reflections I have now. In reading his writings it seemed that I became closer, I can relate, and it seemed that I am very involved. I can read his writing with so much spirit and feeling and I guess, because I like him; I like how he embraces his calling with so much risk and devotion. He is really the man of God, strong and persuasive, true disciple of Christ, a great man. He is truly one of the great pillars of our faith. The following are writings to the different communities and individuals that he wrote after first and foremost thanking God. He was so grateful to the Lord that even though he was an enemy of Christ before and slaughtered many Christians, God never looked on the past but always on his potential to become a true disciple of Christ. He was so thankful to God that in every community he went to, gradually they began understanding the true meaning of being true followers of Christ.

In every letter of St Paul he sent to every community, he never forget to thank God at the very beginning. We called it his "salutation or greetings to the community.

The letter of Paul to the Romans (Rm. 1: 8) - "... *first, I thank my*

God through Jesus Christ for all of you, because your faith is proclaimed throughout the world." 1 Corinthians 1:4- *"I give thanks to my God always for you because of the grace of God that has been given to you in Christ Jesus. For in every way you have been enriched in him, in speech and knowledge of every kind."* 2 Corinthians (1: 3) - *"Blessed be the God and Father of our Lord Jesus Christ, the Father of mercies and the God of all consolation, who consoles us in all our affliction so that we may be able to console those who are in any affliction with the consolation with which we ourselves are consoled by God. For just as the sufferings of Christ are abundant for us so also our consolation is abundant through Christ."* Ephesians (1:3) - *"Blessed be the God and Father of our Lord Jesus Christ, who has blessed us in Christ with every spiritual blessing in the heavenly places, just as He chose us in Christ before the foundation of the world to be holy and blameless before Him in love."*

His letter to the Philippians (1:3) says - *"I thank my God every time I remember you constantly praying with joy in every one of my prayers for all of you, because of your sharing in the gospel from the first day until now. I am confident of this work among you will bring it to completion by the day of Jesus Christ."* Colossians (1: 3) - *"In our prayers for you we always thank God, the Father of our Lord Jesus Christ, for we have heard of your faith in Jesus Christ and of the love that you have for all the saints, because of the hope laid up for you in heaven."* 1 Thessalonians (1: 2 -6) - *"We always give thanks to God for all of you and mention you in our prayers constantly remembering before our God and Father your work of faith and labor of love and steadfastness of hope in our Lord Jesus Christ. For we know, brothers and sisters beloved by God, that He has chosen you, because our message of the gospel came to you not in word only, but also in the power and in the Holy Spirit and with full conviction; just as you know what kind of person we proved to be among you for your take and you became imitators of us and of the Lord, for in spite of persecution you received the word with joy inspired by the Holy Spirit.* " 2 Thessalonians (1:3-4) - *"we must always give thanks to God for you, brothers and sisters as is right, because your faith is growing abundantly, and the love of everyone of you for one another is increasing. Therefore we ourselves boast of your steadfastness and faith during all your persecutions and afflictions that are enduring.* " **2** Letter to Timothy (1: 3) - *"I am grateful to God—whom I worship with a clear conscience, as my ancestors did—when I remember you constantly in my prayers night and day. Recalling your tears I long to see you so that I may be filled with joy."*

St Paul throughout his writing, never stopped thanking God for giving him so many gifts. His humiliation experience persecuting the Christians turned into glorification after his encounter with Christ on his way to Damascus. He never stopped thanking God for all the favors and many blessings that God bestowed on him. I always remember the celebration of Thanksgiving Day here in North America. The Canadian people celebrate during the month of October and the Americans celebrate in the month of November but it is not about the feast; the turkey, the cranberry sauce or in Newfoundland where the Jiggs dinner and peas pudding completes the thanksgiving celebration. I have seen the different foods set on people's tables but it is not the celebration of joy, being together with family and friends, sharing laughter and stories either, it is deeper than that. Although it is not a church Holiday but a Federal Holiday, I guess the President or the Prime Minister wanted to observe the day to thank God. Whatever pleasures they enjoy today, they have come from the bountiful gifts of prosperity and freedom that God showered upon them. They thank God that everything comes from Him and they survive because of God's blessing.

Most of the time, we forget to thank God for the plentiful harvest of goodness, the blessings of the family, blessing of good job and health and we seldom recognize His generosity and kindness. God is so good in so many ways that only the simple heart could tell the way we thank God is to bring back our gratitude and praise His name through our moment of prayer.

We have to be thankful to God not only for the things and blessings we enjoy at this moment but the fact that He loved us so much. We thank God for giving us His only Son to save us from damnation and that is the greatest gift of the Father to us. We always remember that the greatest meal, the greatest thanksgiving, does not happen at our table full of food and wine but in the celebration of the Eucharist. First, He loves us, He died for us, He rose from the dead, that someday, sooner or later He will set a feast for us, a sumptuous feast that we will share with Him forever.

Moreover, every piece of Paul's writings have become my inspiration to write about my own journey at the hospital where I take care of the sick and see how I am able to reach out to the non practicing Catholics there. I like also to tell the people who are in bed to thank God every minute of their lives. They suffer so much, but like St Paul, he also suffered persecution, he was imprisoned and abandoned by some of his friends but he knew very much that Christ, is so faithful, and can't afford to neglect him, for what he is doing is what He has commanded him to do. In our life we should be grateful to God every day, wherever we are, either in the hospital or at home. I never mind going to the hospital every day, I never mind that sometimes I have never had a day off, I never mind if there is a call for the last rite every day, it is my joy to serve these people. I am very grateful, that at the end of the line, I can see on the face of the patient, the happiness and joy for the gift of life that God entrusted to them, that in spite of their worries and pains, they have a total trust and faith that God will make something out of their pain. Life indeed is a celebration of joy no matter what. God is so great to us and we should always be grateful to Him.

STORY

On one of my rounds at the hospital, I was in the Chaplain's office, trying to do the lists of the patients who are and what building I'm going to visit. Suddenly I heard someone knocking on my door and when I opened it, he said "Are you are Catholic priest?" surely, I said "Yes," A man said "Well, my father and his family are in the ICU and he is not doing very well, can you come Father, for the last rite?" I said "Yes, I will be there, in a minute, I'm going to finish the lists then I'll follow you" and he left. When I arrived at the ICU, I saw the three brothers and their sister in the waiting room, the wife was inside then the nurse came out to talk to us and tell us how his situation was right then. When I saw him on the bed, he was restless and was yelling to us; he wanted to break the gadgets attached to his body; the wife was crying and everybody was full of tension inside. I prayed, gave the Anointing of the Sick and prayed for his immediate recovery both in body and spirit but my feeling told me that it seemed that he didn't like my presence there.

The family was very apologetic and in a state of disbelief, for they never heard their father being like that before. He was a very pious man, a member of the Knights of Columbus and very faithful to his Catholic faith, and when I talked to his wife and children, I heard nothing but praise about what a kind and loving father he was and how loving and faithful a husband he was to his wife. When I left him, he was still restless and yelling, and I left his room to visit some other Catholic patients on my list. The following day, I was called by the Anglican Minister who was on call, who said that a patient in ICU was requesting a Catholic priest. I was already in the parking lot of the hospital and had just parked my car because I had just left the other building, but the patient that I was about to visit was sleeping and so

I had to see the new list; there were new patients in that main building. I explained to the Reverend, the Anglican minister, that I was there yesterday, but he was restless. He tried to convince me to go and visit again but in the back of my mind, I had decided already to go to him and see how he was doing. So I went. Still the members of the family were in the waiting room and it seemed that the room was over crowded, then I was informed that some of their family members had come from the mainland.

Only a few of us were allowed to enter and when I saw him on his bed, his wife was so happy about my surprise visit and she said that her husband had requested a Catholic priest, the request coming from his own mouth. I gave him the Sacrament of the Sick, and also this time, a small piece, a very tiny piece of the Body of Christ, for he was not allowed to take solid food. I gave a blessing to the whole family and we sang the Salve Regina together. He was smiling and happy and was glad to hear from the family members of their active involvement in their parish and they were wonderful and loving people. This time the whole family was so happy and very thankful for the Sacrament that I brought, thankful for the man lying on bed, the family he nurtured and glad that he had brought them up to become decent people who have a family of great faith in God. Indeed they must be very grateful. Before I left, the eldest son talked to me about what the doctor told them, that they have to prepare themselves because their father's health is deteriorating. He was not happy about it, but accepted it as his father is already seventy nine years old. They were still hoping for the best and I agree that seventy nine years of age nowadays is still relatively young but he was so happy that this time his dad is submissive to whatever the will of the great Father is for him. He knew how much we must we love Him because He loves more unconditionally and with more love than we can give. Most of the time He is inviting every patient to come back to Him and trust in Him once again, for only in Him can we find rest in our burdens and frustrations.

Only through Him will we see His face at the end of our long journey and be thankful to the One who gave us life.

PRAYER
(PSALM 92: 1-3)
It is good to give thanks to the Lord,
To give praises to your name O Most High;
To declare your steadfast love in the morning,
and your faithfulness by night,
To the music of the lute and the harp,
To the melody of the lyre.
For you O Lord, have made glad by your work;
At the works of your hands I sing for joy.
Amen.

THE HOLY INFANT JESUS

Here I try to establish some of the Infancy narrative accounts of Jesus found in the different Gospels. I tried to establish why millions of people throughout the world including me, are devotees of the Holy Infant, why He touches the heart of everyone. Most of the growing up years of Jesus were hidden. I do believe He grew up like an ordinary child, He cried when He fell down, held the hands of His mom when they crossed in the dark places and He was an obedient child, an inspiration to His parents and neighborhood; full of life and heart to help others. At the very beginning His heart was eager and bursting to help; He did not want to see somebody crying and carrying heavy burdens, He grew up like an ordinary child except when it came to committing sins. In the Gospel of Matthew (2:1-6) it says: *"...in the time of King Herod, after Jesus was born in Bethlehem of Judea, Wise men from the East came to Jerusalem asking, "Where is the child who has been born king of the Jews? For we observed his star at its rising and have come to pay him homage." When King Herod heard this, he was, frightened and all Jerusalem with him, and calling all the chief priests and scribes of the people, he inquired of them where the Messiah was to be born. They told him, "In Bethlehem of Judea; for so it has been written by the prophet": "And you, Bethlehem, in the land of Judah, and by no means least among the rulers of Judah; for from you shall come a ruler who is to shepherd my people Israel."*

And in the Gospel of Luke (2:7) it says: *"...and she gave birth to her firstborn son and wrapped Him in bands of cloth, and laid*

Him in a manger, because there was no place for them in the inn.'
Matthew's Gospel (2: 11-12) states: **"On entering the house, they
(the Wise men) saw the child with Mary His mother and they knelt
down and paid Him homage. Then opening their treasure chests,
they offered Him gifts of gold, frankincense and myrrh.**

And also in Matthew (2: 12-15) it says: "*...and having been
warned in a dream not to return to Herod, they left for their own
country by another road. Now after they have left, an angel of the
Lord appeared to Joseph in a dream and said, "Get up, take the
child and His mother and flee to Egypt and remain there until I
tell you; for Herod is about to search for the child to destroy Him."
Then Joseph got up took the child and His mother by night, and
went to Egypt and remained until the death of Herod.'*

In Matthew (2:19-23) it is related that: "*When Herod died an
angel of the Lord suddenly appeared in a dream to Joseph in
Egypt and said "Get up take the child and His mother, and go to
the land of Israel, for those who are seeking the child's life are
dead." Then, Joseph got up took the child and His mother and
went to the land of Israel. But when he heard that Archelaus was
ruling over Judea in place of his father Herod, he was afraid to
go there, and after being warned in a dream, he went away to the
district of Galilee. There he made his home in a town called
Nazareth, so that what had been spoken through the prophets
might be fulfilled. "He will be called Nazorean."* In Gospel of Luke
(2: 21-24) it states: *Jesus is named and presented in the temple.
"After eight days had passed, it was time to circumcise the child;
and He was called Jesus, the name given by the angel before He
was conceived in the womb. When the time came for their
purification according to the law of Moses, they brought Him up
to Jerusalem to present Him to the Lord (as it is written in the law
of the Lord, Every firstborn male shall be designated as holy to the
Lord) and they offered a sacrifice according to what is stated in*

the law of the Lord, "a pair of turtle doves or two young pigeons."
And according to the law of Exodus (13:1-2) it says: *"The Lord said to Moses: consecrate to me all the firstborn; whatever is the first to open the womb among the Israelites, of human beings and animals, is mine." and that "Every first born, both human beings, and cattle are sacred to Go and therefore, Jesus as the first born was consecrated to God.*

After the boy Jesus was lost and found, in the temple that is, according to Luke (2 ; 41-42) it says: *"When Joseph and Mary went to Jerusalem for the festival of the Passover and when He was twelve years old, they went up as usual for the festival."* Again in the Gospel according to Luke (2:51-52) it says: *"…then He went down with them and came to Nazareth and was obedient to them. His mother treasured all these things in her heart. And Jesus increased in wisdom and in years. And in divine and human favor."* And in Luke (3; 23) it reads: *"When He was thirty years old He began his work.* We heard about His birth in a manger and His purification at the temple when He was eight days old, and then when He was twelve years old and He was lost in the temple and found among the Scribes and Pharisees we heard about Him but after that we never heard or read about Him. His life was not revealed and it is considered the hidden life of Jesus, the untold story of the life of Jesus, and in that we believe that He became obedient to his parents and lived as an ordinary, lovely child when He was that young.

I believe He was loved by everybody for His gentleness and kindness, for His love of his family and His neighborhood and by those who knew Him while He was helping His foster father cut the wood, hammer the nails to make a cabinet or bench, because His foster father Joseph was a carpenter. I would like to dwell on the Infant life of Jesus for a while because His youth and adolescent years were not recorded but His infancy years brought millions of people to conversion and eventually devotion to His name. Yes, millions of people are devotees to the Holy Infant. There were among the few great saints those who were devotees to the Holy Child, like St Francis of Assisi who had his devotion to the mystery of incarnation. He observed the Feast of the Birth of the Infant Jesus with great rejoicing and that's why we have a very festive Christmas celebration, because of him. The Christmas crib of St Francis became the heritage for future generations and it is carried in every corner of the world.

St. Anthony de Padua, following the example of his founder and master, likewise marveled at the Holy Infant Jesus and was often granted the privilege of holding Him in his arms, this being the way St. Anthony is generally depicted by the artist on his statue. It is St. Teresa of Avila, in Spain in the 5000's, Spain's golden Century, who made the Infant known but not only to her fellow Carmelite nuns inside the monastery. In her mysticism St. Teresa found great spiritual benefits in meditating on the Child Jesus and she loved to consider the Child King in the mysteries of the Infancy. Her disciple and co-founder of the reformed branch of the Carmelite Order, the great St John of the Cross, bore such devotion for the mystery of God made man, that he often carried the image of the Child Jesus in procession during the Christmas season.

St. Therese of the Lisieux, one of my favorite saints, was a Carmelite nun and when she entered the convent, she asked to be given the surname of the Child Jesus and the Holy Face and pledged to decorate the statue of the Divine Child in the cloister until death. St. Therese of Lisieux is remembered mainly for her, 'Little way' of spiritual childhood. The Holy Infancy was for her a source of spiritual uplifting. Her 'Little way ' was based on the simplicity and trust of a child in her relationship with God.

And even until now, through her closeness to the Holy Infant, she's still showering roses to those who ask help from her name. Though she is not present physically but spiritually she is everywhere, she is still sending roses as her promise to spend her heaven by doing good here on earth. In her 'Little way', in her little hand she asked the little King to fill up her hands to bring comfort and miracles to the people who asked petitions and miracles. Moreover, the famous Holy Infant Jesus of Prague was originally from Spain. In the 17th century this beautiful statue was brought by a Spanish princess to Bohemia and presented to the Carmelite monastery. For centuries this statue has been enshrined on the side in the church of Our Lady of Victory in the city of Prague, the capital city of the Czech Republic. And even until now His miracles and blessings and cures attract an even increasing number of devotees who worship and appeal to Him in every need.

In the Philippines, the devotion to the Holy Infant, Sto. Nino is celebrated especially in the cities of Cebu. On April 7, 1521, the Portuguese navigator Fernando Magallanes arrived and planted the cross on the shore of Cebu, claiming the new territory in the name of the King of Spain. He presented the image of the Holy Child, the Sto. Nino, as a baptismal gift to Hana Amihan, wife of Raja Humabon. Hara Amihan was later named, Queen Juana in honor of Juana, mother of Carlos 1 and along with the rulers of the island, some 800 natives were also baptized to the Christian faith. At that moment of receiving the image, it was said that Queen Juana danced with joy bearing the image of the Holy Child.

The Augustinian friars that accompanied Miguel Lopez de Legaspi in his expedition proclaimed miracles and built a church on the site where the image of the Holy Child was found. The San Agustin Church was later named the Basilica Minor del Sto. Nino and even until now the millions of devotees of this Holy Child come from different parts of the world. I love this humble little King and that's why I include it here in my book for I am one of his great followers and believers.

Sometimes I think, this Holy Child has never remained a 'child'; He grew, He preached, He died and He resurrected from the dead; and then I think I have missed the point. Well, I may have missed the point, but I have to realize that there is an important point on the "childhood" of Jesus that should not be ignored just as at the same time, there are points and traits in our Children that should not be missed out. The heart of the gospel of Mark (Mk 10:13-16) *says: "People were bringing little children to Him in order that He might teach them; and the disciples spoke sternly to them. But when Jesus saw this, He was indignant and said to them, "Let the little children come to me; do not stop them; for it is such as these that the kingdom of God belongs.*

Truly I tell you, whoever does not receive the kingdom of God as a little child will never enter it." and then He took them up on His arms, laid his hands on them, and blessed them."

Furthermore, certain persons are gifts and I have to thank God for allowing me to know them for they are gift to me. I met Susan Papas Hauck and her husband Larry Hauck during the enthronement of the Holy Infant at the Our Lady of Peace Parish here in Victoria. We were sitting at the same table and after we introduced ourselves to each other we exchanged different views regarding faith and their devotion to the Holy Infant. They invited me to visit their home any time for they live on the mainland of Vancouver. After two months I guess, I went to their home for a particular reason and I was really surprised and amazed at the beautiful Holy Infant's of Prague they have inside their house. The altar was so full of the different sizes of the statues of the Holy Infant and the statue and image of the Blessed Virgin Mary. As I came to know her, she told me how she was very close to the Holy Infant and how when she was young she was already a devotee and she had a little statue that she carried always wherever she went. She prayed through this baby Infant about her dreams and plans for her future life and how she will come to help out families in dire need. She told me they were thirteen siblings and her father died when the youngest was only barely three months old, indeed a difficult time for them to survive and stay together. Seeing with pity, the role of a single parent like her mom, she wanted to help. She never lost hope and she prayed to this Baby Infant that she wanted to work abroad here in Canada to help the whole family.

In short, all her dreams came true and she attributed it all to the help of the little King, the owner of our own destiny. Only three of her siblings are left in the Philippines for they would rather choose to stay there, but the other ten of them are enjoying living here in the beautiful city of Vancouver with their own families and kids. But what she is most thankful for is most of her siblings are very active in the church, very committed to their faith. The value of prayer is still very strong and solid in them. Susan in her own little way wanted the Holy Infant to be known not only in Prague in the Czech Republic and Aranzano, Italy but also here in Vancouver and Vancouver Island. She had a lot of stories of miracles to tell regarding her devotion to the Holy Infant and even until now, she travels to Prague many times just to witness the Feast of the Holy Infant. She has bought many statues and replicas of the Holy Infant of Prague and donated them to the parish. She also likes to dress up the Holy Infant in very fancy clothes and with golden regalia, for she is a dressmaker. In her devotion to Holy Infant, one day is just not enough to listen to her stories of all her encounters with her devotion.

Susan told me once, *"Father, if you have that devotion to the Holy Infant, it will manifest on you; the childlike virtues will be seen in your external actions."* And I certainly agreed with her. The simplicity, honesty and dependability are common traits of what the Holy Infant wants from us. Indeed, the whole family, her husband Larry and daughter Nicole are blessed with simplicity, with devotion, relying only on the providential care of the Holy Little King, and in return on all the kindness and goodness that the Holy Infant showers upon them. She wanted to share and to propagate the devotion to the Holy Infant, to everybody, so that we all experience the wonder, the kindness and the miracle of the Little King. Their devotion to the Holy Infant / Sto. Nino is a reminder for us Christians that it is God's will that we should remain humble children before the eyes of God. Although we grow in age, our values should remain like that of child. In fact, a Holy Child was born in order to remind us of our dependence on God. Despite the resources that we have, we must always long for the need of the mercy and providence of God. Despite the power that we have, we always remain powerless and nothing before the eyes of God. We are all God's beloved children and our hearts and minds before God should be those of little children before the Little King.

PRAYER
PRAYER OF A SICK PERSON
O Most Dear and Sweet Child Jesus,
I know you know my heart and my soul,
Look with mercy and love upon your poor servant,
Who Suffer with so much pains and heartaches.
I beg you to cure and heal me.
You are our Heavenly Doctor, O most Beloved Little King
And I do believe you can do all.
For nothing is impossible in Your Holy Name
I trust my life to you, bless me, heal me and console me.
But If it is your will for the atonement of my sins
and for the greater glory of your Name. Amen

three times:
"Glory be to the Father..."

DEVOTION TO THE BLESSED VIRGIN MARY

'MARY MOTHER OF GOD—'PRAY FOR US'—This prayer always plays at the back of my mind every time I think of the Blessed Virgin Mary, our Mother. And this prayer, brings back the memories of when I was ordained, when the Cantor sang the Litany of the Saints and the six of us, who were about to receive the Order of the Priesthood prostrated in the aisle of the church in front of the altar, to surrender ourselves totally to His care and providence, to fulfill the mission of Christ. This prayer registers so much in my mind; it is so melodic, so vivid and always keeps playing. I never forgot it since then; it became my strength and I felt that her cloak was always protecting me from the shadow of death and any dangers, and that with her help and intervention, I can see the fruits that I was fighting for. '**Holy Mary Mother of God—pray for us.**'

This prayer also became my unspoken anthem wherever I go, especially visiting the sick people in the hospital, because I know, she would do her best to ask a favor from Her Son and I have proven it. I must confess, during my formation years in the seminary, I was so close to her that I can air my sentiments and inner thoughts on her during my moments of doubts and worries. I never missed praying the rosary then. I was so blessed that most of the parishes I was assigned to had exposure to her in the parish during summer time, most of them were named after her. During my Ordination to the Diaconate I was ordained in a parish named after her, Our Lady of Annunciation. She was the first one who received the Good News, and she wanted to share that Good News with me. Before I left the Philippines I served as a guest priest in the Immaculate Conception Parish, the parish where I stayed when I was still a seminarian and when I was a Deacon. This has now become the Cathedral of the Immaculate Conception in Pasig, Philippines.

When I came here to Canada via Newfoundland in the Diocese of Grand Falls, the first assignment I had, I was appointed as an Associate Pastor at the Cathedral of the Immaculate Conception. She is the guiding star of my priesthood, the Mother that never rejects but loves everyone; she would sacrifice herself to accompany us in times of troubles and needs. Remember when she learned that her cousin Elizabeth was pregnant, she went with haste just to be with her? She never thought of the dangers of riding the donkey in the desert, with scorpions and snakes on the road, with the scorching heat of the sun; just to be with her cousin and to attend to her needs.

Mary was so attentive to the needs of the people. Remember the wedding at Cana, when the hosts ran out of wine? Mary, for the first time asked a favor from her Son although it was not the right time for her Son to reveal Himself as Son of God, but because it was the request of His mother, He never thought twice but to grant it. That's the role of Mother Mary, that's why she is so well known as Our Mother of Perpetual Help. Millions of people are flocking to ask her help in times of need and no one is left unaided. She is a great Mother and as I said, I was not even worthy to become a priest of Christ but not because of my devotion to the Blessed Virgin Mary. I figured she would ask her Son to reconsider me, just like she did at the wedding at Cana.

The Song of Mary—the Magnificat served as a link, a memoir in my heart of my seminary life and my ministry in my priesthood now.

This prayer is engraved in my soul to remind me how blessed I am to have a spiritual Mother like her. **Mary's Song of Praise the so-called Magnificat.** In Luke (1: 46-55) Mary said:

"My soul proclaims the greatness of the Lord,
And my spirit rejoices in God my savior,
For He has looked with favor
on His lowly his servant.

From this day all generations will call me blessed;
the Almighty has done great things for me
And holy is His name

He has mercy on those who fear Him
In every generation.
He has shown strength with His arms;
He has scattered the proud in their conceit.

He has cast down the mighty from their thrones
And lifted up the lowly
He has filled the hungry with good things,
And the rich He has sent away empty.

He has come to the help of His servant Israel
For He has remembered His promise of mercy,
The promise He made to our fathers,
To Abraham and his children for ever."

In this **Magnificat,** Mary, while under the inspiration of the Holy Spirit, said "Henceforth, all generations shall call me blessed." One of the messages of the "Beautiful Lady" to Bernadette in the apparition of 2nd of March 1858 said: *"Go and tell the priests that people should come here in procession, and that a chapel should be built here." After more than 150 years since the apparition took over,* *the Immaculate Mother showered bountiful blessings and miracles, healing and conversion throughout the world.*

Many great Popes asked the motherly care of the Blessed Virgin Mary on their Papacy reign, and the Blessed Mary indeed took the hands of every Pope close to the heart of her beloved Son. Pope Pius X11 on May 13, 1942, on his 25th Anniversary of his Episcopal consecration said "The Faithful Virgin never disappointed the trust put on her. She will transform into a formation of graces, physical and spiritual graces, over Portugal, and from there, breaking all frontiers, over the whole church and the entire world." The 2002 Apostolic letter of Pope Paul 11 on the Holy Rosary, **Rosarium Virginis Mariae**, further communicated his Marian focus as he explained how his personal motto "Totus Tuus" was inspired by St. Louis de Monfort's doctrine on the excellence of Marian devotion and total consecration. "Since Mary is of all creatures the one most conformed to Jesus Christ, it follows that among all devotions that which consecrates and conforms a soul to our Lord is devotion to Mary, His Holy Mother, and that the more a soul is consecrated to her the more will it be consecrated to Jesus Christ."

The late Holiness Pope John Paul 11 even credited Our Lady of Fatima for saving his life following the assassination attempt on the Feast of Fatima in 1981. The present Pope, Pope Benedict XIV during his visit in France, celebrated the Holy Mass for the Sick at the Basilica of the Rosary in Lourdes and paid tribute to the capacity of Jesus and Mary to cope with suffering and said "When speech can no longer find the right words, the need arises for a loving presence. We seek then the closeness not only of those who share the same blood or are linked to us by friendship, but also the closeness of those who are intimately bound to us by faith. Who could be more intimate to us than Christ, and his Holy Mother, the Immaculate One."

One example of a good priest whose life and discipline was really shaped by the spirituality of the Blessed Virgin Mary, is my friend and classmate Fr. Roger Poblete; for I knew him very well during our seminary life. He was already a faithful devotee to the Blessed Mother even until now and he attributed his joy and simplicity in serving the remote places in the Diocese of Cornerbrook to being like the Blessed Mother, simple but always having the time and golden heart to offer his simple hands to the people who needed his presence and sense of humor. He might forget some things but not the rosary inside his small pocket wherever he goes. The Blessed Mother indeed loves her priests. The Heavenly Mother always held the hands of the priest and led him to her beloved Son.

Another good priest is again another good friend of mine whom I knew in a very simple way. The three of us were priests, a Portuguese, a Filipino, and a Vietnamese, we really enjoy one another's company and the three of us used to have lunch during our day off, every Monday.

Originally he came from Portugal but lived here in Canada for more than twenty five years. He is the present pastor of Our Lady of Fatima Parish but his simplicity in life draws people closer, not only to the Blessed Virgin Mary but mostly to her Son and not only to the novena to Fatima but mostly to the celebration of the Holy Eucharist. He is a man whose kindness and simplicity are seen in his actions and devotion to his calling. His devotion to the Blessed Virgin Mary also is so simple yet very intimate. Every 13th of May and in October, they always have a special celebration dedicated to the Blessed Mother and his brother priests back in Portugal entrust their priestly ministry and their lives to the care of our motherly Mother. Every priest who wants to be faithful to their priestly life should try to hold the cloak of the Blessed Mother.

Furthermore, Mother Mary is the mother of all the sinners and with her, as a priest, I also asked her every day to be with me always, in my ministry wherever a go; I always ask her for her motherly help and guidance. She is the Mother that no matter how much of a sinner I am she would always be there to stand by my side; a Mother who loves us to the very end and always intercedes for us to come closer to her Son. That is also what I always do every time I visit the sick; at the very end I entrust the sick to the Motherly care and protection of the Blessed Virgin Mary and I believe she would accompany to her Beloved Son, every soul that departs from this pilgrimage and she would do her best to do what she can do for that soul and at the end of my every visit, I always sing the *Salve Regina.*

Salve Regina
Mater mesirecoriae
vita dulcedo
et spes nostra salve
ad te clamamus
exsules filii Hevae
Ad te susperamus, gementes et flentes
in hac lacrimarum valle
Eia Ergo, advocata nostra
illos tuos miserecodes oculos ad nos converte
Et Jesum, benedictum fructum ventris tui,
nobis post hoc exsilium, ostende, O Clemens,
O Pia, O dulcis Virgo Maria. Amen

MEMORARE

Remember, O most gracious Virgin Mary,
never let it be known,
that anyone who fled to your protection,
implored your help, or sought your intercession
was left unaided.
Inspired by this confidence, I fly unto you.
O Virgin of Virgins, my Mother,
to you do I come, before You I stand, sinful and sorrowful.
O mother of the world Incarnate,
despite not my petitions,
but in your mercy hear and answer me,
Amen .

Holy Mary Mother of God—Pray for us.